REIKI HEALING FOR BEGINNERS

Balance Your Chakras and Increase Your Energy

(Learn Reiki Healing and Reduce Stress Through Meditation and Yoga)

Soon Macias

Published by Jackson Denver

Soon Macias

All Rights Reserved

Reiki Healing for Beginners: Balance Your Chakras and Increase Your Energy (Learn Reiki Healing and Reduce Stress Through Meditation and Yoga)

ISBN 978-1-77485-230-9

All rights reserved. No part of this guide may be reproduced in any form without permission in writing from the publisher except in the case of brief quotations embodied in critical articles or reviews.

Legal & Disclaimer

The information contained in this book is not designed to replace or take the place of any form of medicine or professional medical advice. The information in this book has been provided for educational and entertainment purposes only.

The information contained in this book has been compiled from sources deemed reliable, and it is accurate to the best of the Author's knowledge; however, the Author cannot guarantee its accuracy and validity and cannot be held liable for any errors or omissions. Changes are periodically made to this book. You must consult your doctor or get professional medical advice before using any of the suggested remedies, techniques, or information in this book.

Upon using the information contained in this book, you agree to hold harmless the Author from and against any damages, costs, and expenses, including any legal fees potentially resulting from the application of any of the information provided by this guide. This disclaimer applies to any damages or injury caused by the use and application, whether directly or indirectly, of any advice or information presented, whether for breach of contract, tort, negligence, personal injury, criminal intent, or under any other cause of action.

You agree to accept all risks of using the information presented inside this book. You need to consult a professional medical practitioner in order to ensure you are both able and healthy enough to participate in this program.

TABLE OF CONTENTS

INTRODUCTION 1

CHAPTER 1: ANGELIC REIKI BASICS 6

CHAPTER 2: BENEFITS OF REIKI HEALING 11

CHAPTER 3: ABOUT REIKI 32

CHAPTER 4: WHAT ARE THE BENEFITS AND LIMITS OF REIKI? 52

CHAPTER 5: WHAT IS REIKI? 66

CHAPTER 6: HOW TO STAY AT A HIGHER VIBRATION 72

CHAPTER 7: THE SCIENCE BEHIND REIKI 78

CHAPTER 8: HISTORY OF REIKI 102

CHAPTER 9: REIKI ENERGY MASSAGE TREATMENT 109

CHAPTER 10: THE DEFINITION OF REIKI: 113

CHAPTER 11: THE REIKI HEALING TOOL 136

CHAPTER 12: REIKI AND YOUR CHAKRA 142

CHAPTER 13: THE THIRD CHAKRA 148

CHAPTER 14: THE DIFFERENCE BETWEEN REIKI AND ANGELIC REIKI 153

CHAPTER 15: LIFE WITH THREE EYES............................. 159

CHAPTER 16: THE FIVE PHASES OF THE CHI CYCLE 170

CONCLUSION 183

Introduction

Reiki is a system of two words: Rei as well as Ki. Rei means widespread, whereas Ki refers to a flow of vitality or life. According to Reiki vitality healing, there are seven vitality centers, or known as chakras, on the spine of the body. A Reiki healer accomplishes this feat by opening their chakras in the crown to receive vast life energy, and they then direct or center the vitality of their hands towards their patient. It is possible to perform this kind of healing in a specific area or even from the separation.

In recent times, many people are looking for Reiki healing, while they are undergoing different forms of the current drugs. According to the firm instructors of Reiki recovering, the physical, emotional and spiritual well-being is affected when a person's life-stream energy is disturbed or blocked in any way. Reiki is a secure and atypical mending option because it's not intrusive and essentially uses the all-inclusive life force.

Reiki recuperating brings a lot of medical benefits. For instance, it helps in loosening the body of the receiver which assists in relieving stress and anxiety. When the body and the brain aren't as full of stress, the secure structure becomes healthier and body becomes equipped to face illness by itself. Another benefit of Reiki that is being recognized regularly is that it helps with sleep deprivation as well as other sleep-related issues.

This is true, realizing that when the body, psyche , and soul are in a state of relaxation the resting process is regular. Hypertension reduction is another well-known benefit of Reiki along with increased imperativeness and resistance. Another benefit of this alternative treatment method which promotes the development of otherworldly aspects is the increase in the body's frequency of vibration.

In a number of different ways Reiki healing is similar to a back rubs, where the patient is lying on a table that is like tables for back rubs, dressed in a completely clean. The air is also the form of a spa. From the delicate lighting to the music that is played softly and quietly.

The process of healing begins by placing his hands on different areas of the body of the patient. The procedure is carried out with a gentle touch and hands are usually put on the body of the person who is quiet for a couple of minutes. Each healer has their individual strategies, with some performing their hands freely in accordance with the vitality stream of the patient.

In no way is it like the way that a lot of people believe, Reiki mending is not an actual religion, but its influence is significant. The people who profit from this all-encompassing treatment method, come from different religions and societies. Even those who don't believe in Reiki recuperating do gain from it. This implies that, in order for it to be effective, you don't require faith in it.

Are Reiki vitality-based mending of work an actual practice? Here we attempt to address these questions.

Specialists, medical professionals analysts, specialists and other experts have evaluated the effectiveness of Reiki treatment in the midst of endless pain, incapacity and inability and day-to-day work insomnia, dependence on medications. Mental manifestationslike anxiety, anxiety and outrage, as well as trepidation and despair, as well as apathy and the inability to release or adjust have been evaluated before, followed by following the event, treatment. Examining is ongoing within the realms of fibromyalgia DIABETES, AIDS and disease. Therefore most results indicate that Reiki and various manifestations of mending touch therapy are effective treatments that have virtually no negative side effects.

Chapter 1: Angelic Reiki Basics

Together working in tandem with working in conjunction with Angelic Realms, Ascended Masters collective, and Galactic beings Angelic Reiki is a method of healing through sound and consciousness expansion.It's an incredible method for personal development, transformation and preparing for ascending.It's the means of healing that we need of our times.

Angelic Reiki can be described as a powerful healing modality that harnesses the power from the Angelic Realm to manifest healing and harmony on all levels to those receiving their energy healing power.With Angelic Reiki we have the possibility of self-healing and also to send healing to other people locations, people and events close and far.

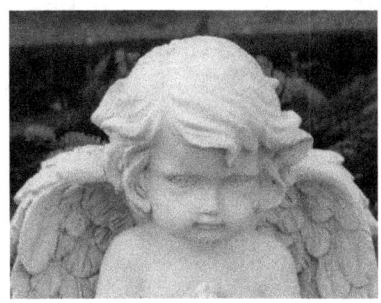

The Basics

Angelic Reiki utilizes the disciplines of The Usui as well as Shamballa lineages and blends them with powerful transmissions channeled by masters.

This is a comprehensive energy healing system that is accessible to all. The attunements prepare and allow individuals to work in partnership together with Angelic Spirits Light and discovered a clear and permanent connection to that Angelic Dimension.

When you receive the Angelic Reiki treatment, the practitioner is simply an intermediary for the healing power of Angelic Reiki to be transferred to the client.

Angels aren't bound to time and space.Working in harmony and working along with Angels and Archangels allows us get deep into all areas that call for the rebalancing of our energy or healing.In Multidimensional Angelic Reiki healing it is the recipient who is helped to release physical emotional, karmic and physical imbalances and the root causes of problems across time and space.It's an honour to share and receive these healing sessions.

The practice for Angel Reiki has the same principles like Usui Reiki.

Archangel Raphael has been called the Angel of Healing however there are many other Angels and Archangels who can help you heal yourself or a situation. Angels are able to heal in a limitless way and can heal emotional and physical suffering. Just ask them for help for healing your own personal pain.

The method for Angel Reiki is the same as Usui Reiki, which is hands off/on as well as remote therapy. One could choose to be seated or lying on a sofa like with all Reiki, and it is completely covered during the treatment. The ambience is created by soothing music that can be extremely beneficial to the treatment and also help the patient to feel more relaxed.

This Angel Reiki energy is channeled into the realm of angels through the assistance from Ascended Master, Archangels and Angels, that is then transmitted via the fingers of the practitioner to the person who wishes to receive healing.

Angels could help us get to the places that need to be addressed, that require healing and balance and allowing us to be surrounded by love and support to release emotional, physical and Karmic imbalances.

Crystals can be utilized to get rid of and heal blockages.

Angel Reiki is soft and affectionate.

The entire process of Reiki is the method that works with a person's energy system. The objective is to eliminate negative energy that is harmful and replace it by harmonious positive and healthy energy.

Chapter 2: Benefits Of Reiki Healing

Reiki is an non-invasive touch therapy for healing which helps improve physical, mental and emotional well-being. It also aids in enhancing spiritual health.

The reduction in stress is among the most significant advantages. In general, people are more at coping with anxiety and stress when at peace with their mind. Stress is linked to many ailments like the heart, high blood pressure cancer and stroke. In a state of calm the immune system activates natural healing capabilities.

Another benefit of reiki for health is the emotional and mental balance which helps improve memory and increase the ability to concentrate. It also aids in improving mental clarity. Regular treatment can improve the mind, improving its clarity and sharpness.

Reiki can also assist in easing the feelings of anger, fear and frustration, and can also help improve mental well-being. Peace and harmony in the inner are powerful instruments for spiritual development. Many claim to feel better and have more restful sleep after having the therapeutic effects of touch.

It has been established that reiki can improve personal relationships by increasing the ability to connect with loved people. It boosts empathy, and can create an emotional connection that lets people bond at a deeper level which makes relationships stronger.

During therapy sessions, emotional issues are remediated and prevented from consuming the mind. It boosts energy and assists in the reduction of depression and anxiety. It also helps reduce mood fluctuations.

Another benefit to health is the reduction of discomfort. The people who go through treatment with touch, report feeling less pain in different areas of the body, including shoulders, arms and legs, as well as the back. Reiki can also help relieve the pain caused by a variety of conditions like migraines, headaches, and arthritis.

It can also help reduce joint inflammation and reduce asthma and fatigue symptoms. Furthermore, it may speed up recovery from a chronic disease or surgery and may reduce side consequences of certain medicines to recover.

Reiki is rapidly becoming a common method of treatment in clinics and hospitals and is among the most efficient and effective ways to improve your overall mental and physical well-being.

HISTORY OF REIKI HEALING

The story of reiki is rooted in the past in Japan. There are numerous stories about it, but it is widely accepted that reiki can be traced all the way back to Dr. Mikao Usui who lived in Japan during the latter part of the 1800s.

Dr. Mikao Usui is believed to have traveled to numerous regions of the globe during his lifetime. He was at one point an Tendi Buddhist Monk. It was at this point when he was more aware of the concept of spiritual healing.

In the same way that as Dr. Usui had traveled before becoming a monk, it is believed that influences from the outside were incorporated into his healing. There are other forms of physical and spiritual healing like Chinese medicine Eastern healing systems such as Chi Gong and the Japanese equivalent Kiko are discovered in what we now call reiki.

Dr. Usui is believed to have been a adept healer and teacher who gained fame quickly across Japan. His first clinic/school was opened at Tokyo around 1922. The methods and teachings included in the spiritual healer's system were effective well for a wide range of illnesses. While his school was primarily to teach spirituality, many received free or low-cost treatment.

Usui The teachings of Sensei were broken down into 6 levels.

In the beginning, Shoden (student) that has four different levels. At this level, the students had to work hard to improve their spirituality. Only after they had mastered this was it possible to move on to the next stage that is Okuden or inner wisdom. According to reports, only a few of his students could pass this stage and moved on to the next level.

The final level is Shinpi-Den or the secret or mysterious instructions. Dr. Usui was believed to have instructed over 2000 individuals. One of those students was Chujiro Hayashi.

Dr. Chujiro Hayashi is thought to be among the few who was able to become masters under Dr. Usui. It is believed that he was the creator of the hand posture system which is still which is still used in the west. Dr. Hayashi employed seven to eight hand positions for treating the upper body. The idea that the torso and head was treating the major centers of energy, which then flowed throughout the body. He could have also adapted other hand positions that are used in reiki the present.

It was in his time as an acupuncturist within Japan when Dr. Hayashi had a patient named Mrs. Takada who had traveled from Hawaii. Mrs. Takada was so impressed by her healing abilities that she was a student under Dr. Hayashi. And when she came back to Hawaii she started a Reiki teaching in Hawaii.

Mrs. Takada was initiated to Reiki master in 1938. She was later initiated to 22 masters.

REIKI ENERGY

The word"reiki" is derived in two Japanese words, namely the words rei and ki.

Rei represents the higher level of intelligence which guides the development of the universe and everything it has to offer. It is able to help us learn more about our universe as well as the environment around us.

Ki is the non-physical energy found in every living thing and not just humans as well as animals, plants and even the environment. If someone has an abundance of ki, they're resilient and are able to take on the challenges they take to with confidence. If someone has a lower ki, they are more prone to diseases.

An individual can boost their ki levels by doing breathing exercises, soaking up plenty of sunlight, and having enough sleep.

If ki and rei are combined Reiki is described as an energy resource that isn't physical, but it has a tremendous healing capabilities through the life-force energy sources controlled by a higher power.

Reiki can't be forced We must locate a space where we can focus on our energies and healing power without getting distracted. Reiki can help us get our minds into an optimal state. Once your mind is healed, your body will begin to heal itself.

Negative energy can be found within the body as well as the mind. The practice of reiki assists the body to regain its balance. Even unhappy and unhappily-thoughts are detrimental to our bodies and, together with any toxins found in the organs and cells, must be removed to reach a tranquil and well-being state.

THE FIVE REIKI PRINCIPLES

Dr. Mikao Usui, who we are familiar with from the chapter about the development of Reiki healing is believed to be as the ancestor of reiki and developed the five reiki principles. It is believed that they originated from the writings of Emperor Meiji who was who was the 122nd Emperor from Japan who reigned between 1852 and 1912.

The secret of attracting joy,

The miracle cure to cure all illnesses.

For today, at least:

Do not be angry.

Be assured,

Be thankful,

Do your best,

Be kind to everyone.

Every day and night Join your hands for meditation and pray from your heart.

Write it down and sing with your mouth.

To improve the body and mind.

Usui Reiki Ryoho.

The person who founded the company,

Mikao Usui.

It is believed that if you adhere to these easy steps, you'll be more calm and healthy life.

AT LEAST FOR TODAY I WILL NOT BE ANGRY

This is a fairly easy thing to say However, in our hectic and hectic lives, practicing it can be a challenge. The personal space we inhabit isn't always one of peace and harmony.

Negative emotions are thought to cause serious blocks within our own energy that affects all aspects of our souls and minds. If we release anger, we can be blessed with the peace of mind and happiness.

AT LEAST FOR TODAY I WILL NOT WORRY

We all worry about our own at some point or another. Certain of us are so adept at living with anxiety that we can no recall what life would be without it.

The burden of filling our hearts and minds with anxiety only eats at our soul and body. There won't be peace or joy in our lives if they are full of anxiety.

If we release the burdens of life the mind is filled peace and calm that leads to inner peace and well-being.

AT LEAST FOR TODAY I WILL BE GRATEFUL

Well-being and happiness is often easier when we appreciate the things in our lives. When we are grateful, our mood increases and we feel happy in our own world.

If we truly feel grateful from the heart, that gratitude will bring more happiness that we feel in our lives.

Giving a thank-you, giving smiles to those who pass by or giving an encouraging words to our fellow citizens are all small things. These little acts can go a long way to make our hearts feel more relaxed and allow us to view things in a positive way.

A smile is free however it gives you an abundance of benefits.

AT LEAST FOR TODAY I WILL DO MY WORK DILIGENTLY

The majority of us make a living to support ourselves and it's a great benefit for us to be satisfied with the work that we are given. When we are able to give our time in a sincere manner, we can feel peace of mind in our lives.

If we are honest and make an effort to treat our jobs or our bosses with respect then only will be able to feel satisfied.

AT LEAST FOR TODAY I WILL BE KIND TO EVERY PERSON I MEET

We all feel that being compassionate is something we do often. However, stress, anxiety and even emotional turmoil can lead us to lose our the focus of how we treat people who are around us.

If we treat with kindness our family, friends, coworkers as well as our elders, and strangers, we experience an inner tranquility.

Being kind can help others to be kind as well. The act of kindness creates a sense of love, which is greatly wanted in the world.

REIKI SYMBOLS AND THEIR MEANINGS

Five symbols are utilized to perform the Usui Reiki Attunement process in which the student's energy levels are increased and the connection to the universe's spiritual energy is enhanced. The initial four symbols are utilized when reiki treatments are performed.

The symbols don't have any particular powers in and of themselves, however they were created as tools to teach for students of reiki to apply when treating and performing attunements. It is the intention the practitioner is using these symbols that activates the symbols.

THE POWER SYMBOL: CHO-KU-REI

Goals: Manifestation, greater power, faster healing as a catalyst to heal

Cho-Ku-Rei can be used to boost the flow of Reiki energy throughout the practitioner, and also increase the healing power.

THE HARMONY SYMBOL: SEI-HEI-KI

The purpose of this is cleansing, protection physical and emotional healing

Sei-HeKi is used to cleanse and purification, as well as protection to cleanse negative energy, and to let go of the spirit of attachment and assist in distant healing.

THE CONNECTION SYMBOL: HON-SHA-ZE-SHO-NEN

The purpose of this is to heal distantly of karma healing and spiritual connection

Hon-Sha-ZeSho transmits reiki across time and space and is utilized in the past, present as well as future health.

THE MASTER SYMBOL: DAI-KO-MYO

The purpose of this program is empowerment Soul healing, empowerment, oneness

Dai-Ko-Myo is an effective healing symbol that can be utilized to cleanse and charge crystals as well as other objects.

THE COMPLETION SYMBOL: RAKU

Purposes: Kundalini healing, chakra alignment

Raku is only used for attunements. It's utilized to open the energy channels of the new healer and also to separate the energy of the master attuning and the new healer.

BASIC REIKI HAND POSITIONS

The goal the purpose of Reiki is to regulate the body's energy to bring back healthy living and enhance one's passion for living. To achieve this it is essential to understand the Reiki hand positions are vital. There are nine hand positions. In this article, we will briefly describe the different positions. are.

In the initial position, your hands will be placed over the face. The palms of hands rest to either side of your face making the appearance of a cup that covers the eyes while the fingers touch the forehead. The touch should be soft, not applying any pressure.

In the second, the hands are placed on the crown and top of your head. The hand's heel is placed on the opposite one of the sides next to the ears, and the fingers resting on the crown of the head.

For the third position hands are put in front of your head. The cross is made by putting the arms together. One hand is placed on the neck's nap, while the other hand is placed on the rear of the head.

The fourth position is concerned with the heart and collarbone. The thumb and fingers on one hand can be joined to create a V, and the neck is kept in this Vshaped position. The other hand is placed between the collarbone and the heart.

The fifth posture is where, the jaw and chin are in the fifth position, jaw and chin are held. Hands are then arranged into a cup where the chin rests. The hands are extended to wrap around the jaw.

The ribs are also included in six positions. One hand is resting on the upper side of the rib-cageand provides assistance towards the elbow. The other hand is placed on the abdomen, with the fingers touching the belly.

The seventh position is concerned with the area of pelvis. Your hands rest on your pelvic bone, with the fingertips in contact with the pelvic area.

Shoulders are at the main focus on the 8th position. While elbows and arms are bent above the head, the hands are placed first on the shoulders' blades. While the elbows are bent, hands are stretched out until they touch the middle of the back.

The ninth position focuses on both the back and sacrum. The hands start by resting lightly upon the back of their lower. They are then lowered into the sacral area.

Restoring balance and energy flow is the main focus of reiki hand postures. It is not required to exert any pressure. Simply a gentle stroke is all that is required to unblock any blockage energy.

REIKI BREATHING TECHNIQUES

The act of breathing is one that most of us don't consider as breathing simply happens without any conscious effort from us. In the world of reiki, the belief is that by using the correct breathing technique, we can help us on the journey towards better health.

The way we breathe affects the entire body from the nervous system and the heart, as well as the digestive system, the muscles as well as sleep energy levels, concentration and memory to mention only some.

A majority of people breathe through their chest, which is not a cost-effective method to breathe since it only utilizes the upper part of the chest and uses more power from the muscles. When we only use the chest for breathing, we can take in more breaths and absorption of less oxygen.

Breathe deeply take it out, let it out and then evaluate the difference in your mood. A lot of us take this approach when we feel exhausted or stressed, without even thinking about it. It is our body's way of telling us that we aren't paying attention to it.

The reiki method of abdominal breathing is a way to take care of our bodies. The deep, effective breathing starts by breathing in the abdomen, and then the body is filled with oxygen. It is vital to our bodies.

The process begins with a clear head and making use of hands in making the entire process become routine. By placing our hands down on the abdomen , we're in a position to assess how effective the technique we are using.

Then, gently and slowly into the inside while exhaling a breath for a total of six.

Hold the position for two.

Release pressure gently and breathe into your lungs for a period of six.

Keep it up for two.

The four steps of press keep and let go are referred to as the unit. After 10 breath units you will feel a sense of calm and peace. The most important aspect to this workout is pressing and release.

Once you've learned the physical aspects you can imagine your body releasing negative energy by breathing out, and the drawing in of positive energy when you breathe in.

Breathing through the reiki technique is not difficult but will require practice since it is a habit of breathing in a relaxed manner without conscious effort. It's worth it to keep practicing because it is beneficial to our well-being. If you are having difficulty doing this Reiki practitioners can assist you in understanding the right technique.

Chapter 3: About Reiki

Reiki is an ancient practice. Reiki is practiced for quite a while. It was the brainchild of Dr. Usui, a dedicated Buddhist who was from Japan who trained more than two thousand people in the Reiki method up to his passing. Reiki can be described as "spiritually controlled Life force energy healing"--a type treatment that is based on the energy fields surrounding the body. There are two roots from which the Japanese words that Reiki originate from. "Rei" which means "Higher Power" and "Ki" which means "life force energy".

What is the reason we are alive? It's because of the life force energy that circulates through the cellular compartments of our bodies. We have a lot of life energy, vitality, and good health if this energy flow is abundant within our body. If not, we are at a possibility of becoming sick. Similar to Energy medicine

This is the premise of Reiki. It was developed in Japan and is beneficial for relaxation and to reduce stress levels. Reiki is a technique that relies on the body to reduce stress levels. Reiki energy is guided by the spiritual laws and is communicated by the placing of hands. The prevailing view in energy medicine suggests that there could be stagnation of energy in the body when there is an injury to the body or an occurrence of emotional discomfort. As time passes, illnesses pop out when these energies are blocked. The energy medicine belief system and philosophy is focused on increasing your energy flow within the body. It is through this, the risk of suffering can be dramatically decreased while relaxation and speed of recovery are made possible.

The practice was introduced across in the U.S. through Hawaii in the 1940s, then to Europe in the late 1980s. Reiki is the energy of life that flows across all living organisms. When we are connected to this healing force, that is the primary source of energy in all humans We can draw in the energy that is needed to heal ourselves and overall well-being. It is possible to assist others. Health is complete whenever the "ki" (energy) is flowing freely and is solid. When energy is weak or blocked, it causes signs of emotional or physical imbalances.

Reiki is available to everyone for use. From children to the elderly Reiki is completely secure and natural. Based on research and the experiences of its users it is successful in battling all kinds of illness and ailments.

Quick Facts

Reiki involves the transfer of energy via hands-laying. It is growing in popularity, despite many critiques.

Over a million Americans in the US are now finding Reiki or a similar treatment beneficial and beneficial to their in terms of health, according to a study from 2007. [1]

Reiki is now being included in the standard hospital program. It has been recommended and professionally offered across Europe and in the US.

Enter "Reiki" into Google and you'll get around one hundred thousand results. This is how well-known it has grown over time.

There have been numerous studies but not all of them which have shown that Reiki can help with the pains of many illnesses.

It Isn't a Religion

The Reiki philosophy isn't similar to any religion since it's not or does not require any form of affiliation. It is to be you. Its true source comes directly from God. There aren't any set rules of faith you must be a part of before you can use it. There is no dogmas. Some believe that having a calm or self-assured mindset is an additional benefit to being adept at using Reiki properly, however, that is not the case. You don't need anything to be skilled, believe and confidence in values and so on.

Although it's not an actual faith-based religion Reiki will tell you that need to be living your life with the awareness of certain fundamental ethical guidelines. Peace and harmony with others are essential. That is how you live your life. There are some ethical principles that are universal across all cultures, that Mikao Usui, the Reiki founder--suggested that everyone follow to get the most of this wonderful method.

A Bit of History

The energy system of the body had to be comprehended. The information gleaned from it is the catalyst for Mikao Usui's interpretation of Reiki. He wasn't the person who invented it. He had discovered it. The original practice and method was discovered by Usui from Japan after it was transferred through India into China as well as Tibet.

Everything in Reiki was centered around this legendary man named Mikao Usui. He received a solid education since his parents were part of the upper class. He was devoted from the age of seven to study. This attitude allowed him to learn a lot in his early his life. He was able to master Kiko or Chi-Kung. He also learned to effectively use the sword. He was so passionate and committed that he was willing to read anything that offered a glimpse to how the human body functions. This made him extremely interested in everything that could be learned in the fields of psychology, medicine and theology in his broad and costly education. A few days later, the course of his entire life changed. The question was to an of his pupils during the time being a teacher at an institution of higher learning. The question was how did Jesus be the source of all the miracles that were reported about him and the multitude of sick people he treated? This question was strange.

The question had sown seeds and he began the right path to answer. It turned out to be the catalyst that led him to do the most determined investigation. He was not the type to be hesitant about something that is a mystery. Students claimed they were too young to believe it, and they required evidence. Soon after, he resigned his job at the college and went into the wilderness to seek the answers. The possibility of healing oneself and others will not be a stray from the light of his eyes. That was his fervent passion.

Then off to the holy mountain that are the home of Kori Yama. He fasted there for a at least 21 days. He also meditated for 21 days. The need for meditation was because it could speed up the receptivity of healing energy. It would elevate him to an unimaginable state of consciousness, he believed. In the early day's 21st the anger was starting to build up. Then, just when he was about quit in deep disappointment the energy of a spiritual force flowed over him. In a flash, he was consciously and enlightened. Another benefit he received was the ability to heal , referred to as "Reiki Ryoho". He was in a position to heal his damaged toe within a matter of minutes when he rubbed his hands over it.

The realization that something important was happening and that he was now on the path to a prosperous life, he went back home to his monastic community. After a short time, the monk took his understanding to the slums in Kyoto which are brimming with beggars. For seven years, he lived in the slums taking care of their ailments and attending to their various ailments. While he treated and recovering their health as well as teaching people in the Reiki way of masters. The Dr. Chujiro Hayashi, a retired naval officer and surgeon, was among the twenty or so notable ones he passed the knowledge torch to. For the past ten months, he studied under the guidance of Usui before his passing in the month of March 1926. It was to be the one who further popularized the Reiki method.

"Dr. Hayashi was the next important thing to happen in Reiki's history. Reiki. After mastering Usui's method the first thing he did was establish the first Reiki Clinic in Kyoto. The clinic was attended by a lot of people, both middle class and the lower classes, and remained open until 1940. It offered healing to a lot of people, and was perceived by the general public as a thing, not just a an affluent, but also a successful. His legacy was the development of a completely new Reiki style, but still in the Usui tradition, just some notable enhancements. Hands were added to the style so that every part of the body is covered. Many others were Reiki teachers under his direction due to his new system that made it possible to teach numerous people at the same time. Similar to how he taught Usui There was a second named Hawayo Takata, a woman who picked the concept and taught it throughout all of the United States and the West in general.

Her entry in the world of Reiki the past was somewhat accidental. She was a beneficiary who later became a master. In a certain point of her journey, she made the decision to go to Japan because of the frequent problems regarding her health. She was suffering from a lot of health issues, slowly and believed that a surgical procedure was the best choice to treat her gallstones and appendicitis problems. While in Japan she believed that she may not require a procedure again and decided to determine if there was an alternative to conventional medicine. The name that came to mind of the person she sought advice from was a particular Doctor. Hayashi. At first, she was scared and confused regarding what alternative treatment such as Reiki could possibly do for her chronic health issues She eventually gave in and reaping the benefits within a short time. Her health returned after a few weeks of intense Reiki session with Hayashi. Astonished, she asked to learn how to transfer Reiki energy into others in order that she could be of assistance. The two parties came to an agreement, between 1936 and 1938. During this time she studied the first and second levels of Reiki under the guidance of Hayashi.

After having completed her work with Japan that was one of her home countries and the other was the US She brought Reiki back to her home country. In the ensuing time it was that the West was inundated with this method of healing which is effective in ways that are completely convincing. To increase her effectiveness she enticed Hayashi to to her in Hawaii since she had just opened an Reiki clinic. Hayashi agreed, as she was one of his favorite among the 13 who he attuned. He then introduced her to the third level of Reiki. Masters began to study at her feet in the year 1970 as she began to make small tweaks to the general Reiki system. On the 11th day of December, 1980 she passed away. Her legacy to generations following her was 22 Reiki masters who were well-trained and sound They were the first to be the torchbearers for the technique , and are in turn, responsible for the technique's expansion across the globe to this day.

What Is A Typical Reiki Session Like?

Reiki is nothing less than an incredible miracle as it is described by those who have experienced it. The powerful impact of a Reiki session can help the body clear an accumulation of tension and stress. Additionally, there are four healing effects of Reiki: physical emotional, mental, and spiritual. It's like having the sensation of a thrilling, magnificent feeling of a soothing glow that radiates that radiates from the top of your head down to the soles on your toes. In the surrounding, you feel as if you are enveloped in an enchanted halo and blissful health.

An actual Reiki sessions are always an exciting experience. It's not limited to a specific location or place. It can be performed anywhere insofar as it is peaceful and full of the spirit of friendship. The process begins with the patient wearing all of his clothes on while they sit on tables. A comfy chair is extremely frequent. A soothing, soul-lifting song can be played underneath however it is dependent on the individual's preferences. The 60-90 minute session will always provide an opportunity for the client to share issues he or she is facing and discuss their anticipated outcomes.

The actual treatment is systematic and the practitioner starts with a variety of hand forms across the person. The time per body part will vary from two to five minutes in accordance with the needs of the patient. If there are burns or injuries to the patient The hands of the Reiki practitioner are kept close to the location concerned. Although it is true that the Reiki practitioners hands rest placed slightly above the body of the patient however the actual transfer of energy is carried out by the body of the patient. The hands can experience the sensation of tingling or warmth and they remain in their position until the energy is deemed to be flowing again. The stop can result in a sensation to your hands, and this happens when hands are removed from the area and then placed on another and the process continues.

Reiki Techniques

It is the only Reiki however there is variations in the methods used. Some practitioners use crystals. Some use energy healing tools such as chakra wands. The benefit of these tools is that the practitioners discover that they also allow healing and can be an appropriate negative energy protection option for home owners. In Medical News Today, Annie Harrington Chair of the Reiki Federation of the United Kingdom (U.K) stated:

"Reiki relies on no other instruments beyond the practitioner. We do not use crystals, powders or wands as a general rule. However, one of the benefits of Reiki healing is distance healing (where Reiki is sent over several miles) then, many practitioners will use crystals to assist with the energy vibrations."

The techniques employed by a Reiki practitioner include:

Extracting Harmful Energies

Beaming

Infusing

Centering

Smoothing and Raking the Aura

Clearing

Health Benefits

Professionals with a deep understanding of the concept and application of Reiki reveal that current techniques of science are not able to gauge the life force energy that flows through our bodies. It is only experienced by people who remain in tune with it. In the end, Reiki is proven to help the body's healing process in a way that is completely natural. Alongside the peace Reiki gives, which is well-known as well, it can assist in helping the body reach a state of complete health and overall well-being physically, mentally as well as emotionally. Based on a study from University of Minnesota, University of Minnesota, some of the testimonials that are common to those who've experienced the magic of Reiki sessions, revolve around:

wonderful relaxation and peace

disappearing headaches after sessions

mental clarity

Focused senses

Higher concentration levels

and the feeling of a peaceful night's sleep.

"Intensely relaxing" was the term used to describe the significant benefits that people receive when they took part in Reiki according to an investigation. Other studies have confirmed that it was able to aid a significant amount in helping patients deal with challenges. It also helped relieve anxiety and stress, and helped them keep their overall well-being up a notch. Perhaps due to its relaxing effects on the body, that's the reason cancer patients can claim to feel better when they receive Reiki. The research of Cancer Research U.K deduced that patients with cancer feel better since Reiki practitioners are more attentive to them. Reiki practitioner spends more time with them and, of course, they touch the patients. Certain patients are stressed out; some because of fear of the chemotherapy. The pressure used during Reiki can help a lot.

A lot of cancer patients have experienced relief with Reiki's touching, as have people suffering from chronic pains as well as infertility, fatigue, and pain patterns, and many more. Numerous neurological-related illnesses like Alzheimer Cohn's disease and autism, as well as neuro-degenerative diseases can also be helped with Reiki treatments.

Becoming a Reiki Practitioner

"Attunement" is the name given to the moment when a person is initiated into Reiki as an instructor. It's a completely spiritual experience, and so effective, and it's the moment when the student receives the whole package of the master. What's transferred from the experience, from master from student to master, are attunement energy as well as healing techniques. The process of learning Reiki is easy and free of any type of retraining, whether personal or otherwise. It is not necessary to have any prior training and no set of beliefs and no formal education is required and no knowledge or experience is required.

The majority of the lessons students receive from the various types of Reiki instruction available in the world is based on three main elements that are:

the ethics of the relationship between a practitioner and a client

Understanding and knowledge of the energetics that surround the body

and focusing on learning to master the healing energy.

There are a set of preparations to are required prior to the Reiki attunement process. The fasting period of 2-3 days is an essential element and so is meditation. There are also factors that are connected with nature-based meditation and the release of negative emotions. In general, there are three levels of Reiki and each one has its importance. Only those who have reached the Master level are able to teach others and heal distances, just like the way it works in the prayers of Christianity.

Chapter 4: What Are The Benefits And Limits Of Reiki?

Reiki helps to build it, rebalance and replenish the life force in the person.

Below is a list of a few of the most significant benefits that Reiki offers its users:

* Pain-free , pain-free lifestyle

* Greater mobility and less chance of developing arthritic conditions.

* Minimization, and possibly elimination, of anxiety and stress

* Stabilized heart rate

* Healthy blood pressure levels

* Increased levels of resistance to illness

* Aids in overcoming the adverse side effects that can be a result of chemotherapy

* Improves emotional well-being

Positive outlook

Increases vitality exponentially

* Helps to restore balance to the energy centres (chakras)

Energy levels that are healthy and flow to all organs, muscles, nerves, as well as bones

* Reduction in fatigue

* A lower risk of insomnia

* Greater ability to adapt to changes

• Assists with recovery from addiction or alcohol.

* Focus on the issue

* Calmness in dealing with stress-inducing situations

There are a myriad of advantages that Reiki can provide.

It is crucial to keep in mind the fact that Reiki is not an alternative to modern medical treatment. Also, it is not a healing system incompatible with modern medical practices.

Everyone are able to benefit from Reiki Our children, our parents , grandparents, and even our animals.

Reiki for All Life Stages

Whatever the individual's needs, Reiki normally can provide the solution that is able to be adapted to the needs of a person's life.

Reiki During Pregnancy

Reiki is beneficial for anyone of any age, and even those who are not yet born. Women who are pregnant who practice Reiki can express their gratitude to their baby by placing their hands on their stomach. In doing this they can help mothers let the Reiki energies , which are abundant in them to flow to their infant.

Certain Reiki practitioners consider that, if a mother does Reiki then the baby will also be in a vibrational align with the energy of Reiki as well. It means that a child may get the blessings that Reiki can provide and set it up for a wonderful and healthy existence - a perfect present for any mother to gift her child!

Reiki for Children

Reiki is an effective healing method that is not invasive. This makes it a fantastic option for children, as it allows you to assist them in dealing with the growing difficulties they face (physical as well as emotionally) in a manner that is gentle on the child as well as you.

It's been observed that kids are quite open to the positive effects of Reiki and generally accept the process of Reiki without much resistance.

Treatments for kids are provided exactly the same way as the adult treatments are. The Reiki hand positions are similar but the sessions are less lengthy. This is due to the fact that Reiki energy moves through children faster than it does through adults. Children are not afflicted by the emotional blocks that adults suffer from, which leads to a more rapid, efficient Reiki session.

Attuning Children

While babies are able to be tuned into Reiki but they are not able to use it in a meaningful way. This is due to the fact that the practice of Reiki is more than receiving energy (something babies are great in). Reiki can only be effective requires maturity and a clear intention. Therefore, children who are less than six years old typically are not able to engage in Reiki.

But, children who are older than that, usually between the ages of five and twelve, will not only be aligned to Reiki and Reiki, but they can also use it successfully as well. Through practice, supervision and dedication children in this age group can (often more easily as an adult) be attuned successfully towards Reiki the level of 1. (there are more details information on the Reiki levels in the future book).

It is important to keep in mind that those who are practicing Reiki must be taught to never lay their hands on their non-initiated students. It is because children who don't practice Reiki are likely to be uninitiated and unkind, and are likely to be scared of having a child lay their hands on them. This fear could cause blocks in the energy of both the Reiki practicing child as well as the one receiving the Reiki.

Reiki practitioners must be encouraged and encouraged to practise Reiki on themselves, their stuffed animals, their siblings, and their pets. In the next section doing Reiki with pets can be not a risk since animals are tuned to the energy they will accept or not. Thus the practice of letting your child do Reiki for your pet can be an essentially safe procedure.

Reiki for Seniors

Reiki is certainly appropriate for all different ages. However, since Reiki is especially effective at helping to ease pain, those who are elderly are more inclined to practice the healing practice.

Alzheimer patients (a group that includes the majority of senior citizens) are the most receptive people to Reiki. This is astounding because of their ailments, Alzheimer patients normally find it nearly impossible to use alternative treatments.

However, Reiki allows these types of patients to tap into the healing powers of the art in such a simple manner that the mental blockages of the illness are second to nothing.

As children mature and grow as they get older, they naturally less dependent on their parents or guardians.

This freedom is healthy and natural, as a result of development.

If, however, an adult young or middle-aged person is struck by a condition or illness that deprives the person of their independence and causes them to seek out help as they can't manage by themselves and face this challenge, they do so with a reluctance.

They would feign opposition to the circumstance, making comments such as "I can manage," or "I'm ok." The loss of independence is typically an anxiety that results in certain people not seeking medical help until the situation has reached a point that is beyond the point of needing help.

Many older individuals, however, realize that they will no longer be independently. They are aware and accept the reality that their lives will be much easier with assistance as opposed to without.

Reiki and Pets

The number of pet owners who opt for alternative therapies for their pets is increasing. A growing number of people are turning away from the sole reliance on vets and are instead choosing to seek out therapies like Reiki, Shiatsu, etc.

Animal people are extremely sensitive to their pets as well as their diseases. They want to find treatments that not only keep their pets healthy as well as preventative.

Reiki can be a wonderful solution to this need and provide a powerful treatment that provides holistic results.

By using the energy techniques that are a part of Reiki animals are efficiently and quickly healed, and the possibility of negative side effects is virtually zero. Most of the time, when it comes to animals and Reiki when an animal is exhausted to be healed, they'll initiate an end to the session by simply walking out.

Here's the way in which Reiki can benefit animals:

* Increases the healing rate of physical injuries.

* Relieves stress for the animal

The practice of energy creates an emotional connection between the animal and its the owner, which improves the bond between them.

Haters and Skeptics

Like every new endeavor on the road, whenever we begin with a new endeavor, we're not just in doubt, but we often face the doubts of others as well.

Most of the time it is the doubts of others that may cause us to abandon the new venture, more then our doubts.

My suggestion for you in relation to this is to focus on an eye for. Pick a goal (like the practice of Reiki) and concentrate on that only. Don't allow the opinions of other people to distract you from your goal. Learn the art, practice your skills, and only then will you or should you actually begin to study things.

Reiki Responds Uniquely to Each Individual

Reiki does not have the distinction of a method which discriminates. It is a system that treats imbalance.

There are many benefits from Reiki However, the outcomes of treatment can differ because of a number of variables:

* How many sessions or treatments or sessions Reiki did the person receiving Reiki partake in?

What stage of disease was the person in prior to initiation of Reiki?

* Did the client enter the process with expectations that were either unrealistic or high?

* How open was the person receiving Reiki to help their body?

Belief and Receptivity

Reiki is effective regardless of whether one is a believer in the concept. It works due to its universal laws of energy - laws similar to those of gravity, can't be broken.

But, if someone does not have a desire to Reiki in any way, form or form, the healing and energy associated with Reiki are likely to have a difficult to penetrate the barriers in the person. This is for why many people who believe that Reiki can work eventually are disappointed, particularly when Reiki does not seem to have any influence on them.

On the other hand one hand, a skeptical person who may not even be aware of the Reiki system could nevertheless take a stab at Reiki and experience massive advantages, simply because subconsciously they were prepared to be a recipient of Reiki.

Reiki Benefits Everyone

Whatever your origins no matter where you are from Reiki can help you.

It is a technique that Reiki isn't a skill that is reserved for only those who are wealthy, educated or spiritually mature. Reiki is accessible to everyone who is willing to be open to the Reiki system. The only cost is believing in yourself and accepting Reiki into your life.

Treating Root Causes

Reiki is a technique that must be used continuously. If it is used in a hurry it will only result in immediate effects from healing. To reap long-lasting benefits, the healing system of Reiki is required to be continuously applied.

Benefits of Reiki

Reiki can help you by giving you the power to be more effective by empowering you in the following ways:

* Reiki helps reduce anxiety

* Stress, which can be a source of long-term suffering is a thing that can be eliminated with the application of Reiki

* Reiki is an effective alternative to other traditional health practices.

* Reiki allows food to be cleansed prior to eating them by removing the energy of the food we eat.

* Reiki energy can be effective in helping people manage grief

* Reiki is both healing and helps us heal our emotional scars

* Reiki helps us let off the negatives of life - wounds, people and negative experiences

* Reiki aids us in effectively manifest. This makes it an excellent system for setting goals and reaching

Chapter 5: What Is Reiki?

This is perhaps the most difficult to answer of all. The simple answer is...

Reiki can be described as an ancient type of healing that is believed to have spread throughout Tibet, China and India. It was discovered again in the latter part of the 19th century through Sanskrit doctrines taught from Doctor. Mikao Usui, a Japanese Christian minister and theology instructor. The term Reiki is Japanese is a word that means "Universal Life Energy", similar to"Universal Life Energy" or the Chinese "Chi" or the Indian "Prana". Reiki is the vital energy that is a part of all living things and can be activated in the pursuit of healing. It works at all levels: physical, spiritual, and emotional. Although it is rooted in the ancient Buddhist principles, Reiki is not a religion or a religion. It is a healing method...

However, this is merely an example of a dictionary definition. The analogy below might be more appropriate but it's restricted. Imagine you wake up in a room that is a bit spooky. everything is dark because shutters or curtains are heavy and are covering the windows. Nature calls , and you're required to locate the toilet. You wake up and then you crash onto a desk, shaking contents in a frenzied manner and causing pain to your knee. Due to the dark, it's difficult to figure out the way to get to get around. The space seems vast and threatening. Strange forms loom from the darkness while your imagination is triggered by the late-night movies and half-remembered dreams. You're not losing control, but the pressure inside your bladder is being visible. You must locate that light-bulb. After a few more crashes about , you'll find it and turn to turn on the lights. The simple act alters everything you see. You are able to quickly locate the door open, turn on the lights, and then do what needs to be done. You can recognize the dark-colored shapes for what they are , and when you look at your clock, you realize that it's earlier than you thought. Upon closing the shutters, you are presented with bright, shining morning. All you had to do was press down on a tiny piece of plastic and the world changed in a remarkable manner. You didn't need to be aware of how electricity is created or the way electricity works. All you had to know was that in order to receive light, you need to push downwards on the button. Someone else had already done the work for you before you. If you're feeling the need to investigate, do it! electricity, but it will not allow the light to come on faster or more effectively. Knowing how to use the light in getting the most value from it. To achieve this, there are a few aspects you should know: the existence of an electrical system for lighting at all and what you should do if the light isn't functioning properly and who to call. If you've never experienced the electric light before, you must be shown the basics, but once you've been you have been shown, it won't take long before you're switching light on or off using the finest of them. At first, you might think that it's magical, but it's not the kind of magic that is performed better by specially people or people who wear special clothing and sing some special songs. Anyone can turn on a light whenever they'd like to. It's simple. The possibilities for what you can do with the light is limitless however, it is possible to remain as you are in darkness. It's your choice. Consider Reiki as a switch. It lets you know what's wrong and the person you are and how you might improve your life to fix it and how to go about it. This is only the beginning. What you do next is up to you.

The Reiki Attunements.

The core of the first Degree Reiki course is in the attunements (also called initiations) that you receive. In these sessions workshops, your physical and spiritual body will be tuned to be open as well as your energetic system (also called your chakras) is aligned to channel and receive Reiki which is which is the Universal Life Force, by the use of an ancient technique learned by the Dr. Usui.

Once you have received an attunement for the first time, you will feel energy flow through your hands with the notion of healing. The last attunement seals the empowerment so that your channels remain open throughout the remainder of your life. Once you've attuned, the power to heal does not disappear even if not utilized for a long time.

In the Second Degree, you will be given a further two attunements. The reasons behind these attunements will be looked into in a future time.

When you graduate, an additional attunement is offered.

There's not enough space within a compact volume such as this one to discuss the specifics of the attunements. Neither is it the appropriate place.

They are the only necessary attunements to practice Reiki.

Chapter 6: How To Stay At A Higher Vibration

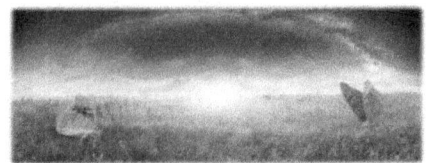

Change comes from the moment Reiki is introduced into your life. The more you let changes to happen and are able to accept it the simpler it will be. Change happens best when you go with the current of changes and allow instead of taking a dive into the current and trying to fight every change that is beneficial to you. A major and popular changes that come when you practice Reiki is the alteration of your frequency within the Universe. Most of the time, following each Reiki attunement, you'll be moved into a different level of vibration, however it can occur at any time.

If you are manifesting, one of the most crucial steps is to let yourself believe that you already have what you want. You are actually experiencing the vibrational level of whatever you desire. It is necessary to transmit the vibration in order to receive the energy.

A higher vibrational level indicates that you are operating at a higher positive frequency and radiating positivity and goodwill to the world around you. Positive energy flows into your life more freely and it's less likely to cause you trouble. People refer to the process of raising an energy level as moving closer to awakening. One interesting thing I've read over and experienced in my own experience is that prior to or following the move up the vibrational level, you might be feeling like you're craving protein. The theory is that it happens because your body requires the additional energy needed to take the leap to a higher level. You might also notice that you're suddenly in need of more sleep

, out of the blue or that you're trying to get rid of material possessions or items from different aspects in your daily life which don't are suitable for you. If you experience some of these things, you should you should know that it's typical and that you're not all on your own. These are all normal actions in an incredibly complex process.

When you reach the new vibration, you must continue to live the right way in order to remain in the higher level. Of course, moderation throughout your life is crucial, but it is essential to keep a healthy, balanced life style to aid in your journey upwards on the vibrational ladder.

Methods to get towards or remain at a higher frequency:

Reiki treatments (from other people and/or self-reiki daily)

Refraining from doing anything that doesn't serve you

Let the things that don't work in every aspect of your life will naturally fall away

You can surround yourself with positive energy

Consume a balanced diet of vegetables and fruits, and If you're an animal lover, take note of the way in which animals were treated prior to and after being killed. This could have an effect on the vibratory levels of the meat you consume. Additionally, fish and chicken are more vibrational that red meat. One rule to follow is that if the meat has hooves, it's lower vibration to consume.

Enjoy uplifting music

Get up and dance around your home... Get loose

Participate in any exercise that make you smile on your face

Exercise

Laugh

Let the sun shine on your skin

Meditate

Keep a note in your journal of the ways that different people and things can affect your feelings.

If you have to express something, say it. Don't hold your emotions inside. If you're not comfortable talking to someone about something, take a note on an article of paper and then wait for several days. The earlier you write it down, the more effective.

Salt baths

Keep crystals and stones with high vibrations around you like quartz and tanzanite.

This is a list that's general for all people, but the one I would recommend is to keep a diary for a couple of weeks and note down every little things that makes you joyful or sad. If it doesn't make you feel happy, it should be removed! It will have incredible impacts on all areas of your life. This will aid Reiki in bringing only the best happiness to your life. I wish you happiness and love

Chapter 7: The Science Behind Reiki

Reiki is an example of an aspect of vitalism, which is the belief of a pre-logical nature that powerful vitality is able to speed up the life and is the factor that separates life-forms from other living objects. The concept of vitalism has always been an academic place-holder, and was responsible for whatever aspects of science weren't yet understood. As science progressed eventually, we were able to comprehend the vast majority of the fundamental aspects of our existence and there was there was nothing for the basic power to accomplish. The power, as such, became a mystery to logic. This is not to mention the fact that nobody has ever been able to prove the existence of an important power, and it is mysterious to scientists.

However it is, the demise of superstition and science from the past has become what is the "elective medication" of today.

There are a few supposed "CAM" modalities that depend on vitalism, such as Reiki. Reiki is, in reality is basically the same as therapeutic contact, which is another method of healing vitality that was common in the medical field even though it is true that it continues to be employed, it's a lot less popular after a multi-year old lady (Emily Rosa) carried out a thorough study to prove that it was merely self-double handling. Reiki is a pleasant way to fill in the gap.

The test of Reiki and healing of the vital organs after all is said and performed is similar to that of many other modalities, all with a very low logical credibilities that are not given enough attention by medicinal researchers. The study is of mostly low-quality small, poorly controlled tests which appear designed to validate Reiki instead of determining whether it is effective. The most recent conducted studies, for example it reveals a high level of anxiety and self-detailed growth in patients with malignancies and concludes that patients feel more comfortable when they are given the attention of a medical professional. The exam is completely ineffective, and consequently is of doubtful value. It is important to think about this exam, which is a complete effort in futility and exhaustion and effort, since the outcome was not in doubt.

A review of 2011's Reiki concentrators was concluded:

The research currently available doesn't allow endings in the efficacy or effectiveness of the process of recuperating vitality. The future research should adhere to the current standards of research into the effectiveness and effectiveness of treatment and considering the mind-blowing character of the potential outcomes the possibility of cross-disciplinary approaches could be crucial. In order to expand the scope of preclinical studies Psychosocial interventions should be analyzed and studied rather than dismissed as untrue treatment

Reiki (articulated Ray-Key) is a kind of "vitality recuperating," basically the Asian variation of confidence healing or the laying on of hands. Experts believe that they bring vitality into the patient, thereby increasing their potential. The education is well-known by medical professionals, and is actually refined by my foundation's attendants (Yale).

Reiki is an ancient Japanese technique for reducing stress and unwinding which further aids healing. When the "life power vitality" is low, we're likely to get sick or feel pressure, or in the event that it's elevated it is progressively a good sign that we are well-equipped and healthy.

Reiki is, in this way, one of the forms of vitalism. It is the pre-logical belief that some spiritual energy is vital to the living. It is the element that separates life-forms from other living ones. The concept of vitalism has always been an academic place-holder, and was responsible for whatever aspects of science weren't yet understood. However the advancement of science over time, we figured out the major aspects of our lives and there was essentially no more for power of nature to perform. In this way, it was able to separate from logic. It is possible to add the fact that no one had the opportunity to prove the existence of an important power - it is completely unresolved to science.

It is true that the dissolution of superstition and science of the past has become an "elective prescription" of today. There are various alleged "CAM" modalities that depend on vitalism, such as Reiki. Reiki actually is basically the same as therapeutic contact, a different method of healing vitality which was widely known to medical professionals, but even though it is still used, it has become less popular after a young multi-year-old woman (Emily

Rosa) carried out an incredible study to prove that it was self-misdirection. Reiki was able to fill in the gap.

The research on Reiki and the healing of vitality when all said and completed, is similar to that of many other similar modalities, ones with a low level of credibilities in terms of logic that aren't considered by medical researchers. The study is mostly low-quality tiny, uncontrolled studies which appear to be designed to validate Reiki rather than to determine whether it actually works. The most recent conducted examination, for instance examines the level of nervousness and self-detailed growth in malignant patients and concludes that patients feel more relaxed when they receive the loving support of a medical caregiver. The examination is not controlled and is not worth the money. You should think carefully about this investigation, which is a total effort that is futile and ineffective since the outcome was not in doubt.

The research currently available doesn't allow any conclusions about the feasibility or the quality of the vitality repair. The future research should adhere to the existing standards of research into the effectiveness and efficacy of treatment. Considering the complex character of the potential outcomes Cross-disciplinary approaches could be crucial. To extend the reach of the clinical preliminary tests Psychosocial processes should be studied and evaluated instead of being dismissed as fake treatments.

The current exploration is of such poor quality that we are unable to draw any useful conclusion from it. Although I don't agree, which essentially means that further research is needed. The lack of credibility of using the mystical power that has not been proved to be present by medical science suggests something else. The last paragraph is strange - it implies that the authors are trying to convert fake effects into actual ones. This is increasingly the practice of a few drug advocates who are elective, in order to be certain that the majority of the treatments they advocate aren't in a way that is superior to fake treatment (which implies they aren't effective).

Reiki is currently within that group. The report, which was distributed at roughly the same time to the audit (and as such, was not included from the study) is a meticulously planned investigation of Reiki in which Reiki was compared to fraudulent treatment Reiki (somebody who is not trained to practice Reiki is essentially making an imsincere effort) in contrast to normal consideration (no mediation). It is not surprising that both the real Reiki as well as the fake Reiki gatherings showed greater self-revealed success than the no mediation group, but they were not distinct from each other. This is because Reiki was not superior to fake treatments.

This means that Reiki isn't effective (at at all within the realm of a scientifically-backed prescription).

Reiki (articulated Ray-Key) is a form of "vitality recuperating," basically the Asian method of repairing confidence or the laying on of hands. Practitioners recognize that they are bringing vitality into the person which increases their financial success. The education is widely accepted by healthcare professionals and is essentially refined by my personal assistants at my personal organization (Yale).

Reiki is an Japanese technique for stress reduction and unwinding. It also aids in healing.

Reiki is, therefore, a kind of vitalism, the belief that an supernatural energy is able to energize the living and is the element that separates living from non-living objects. The concept of vitalism was always an academic position-holder in control of the parts of science that were not yet understood. In the end the advancement of science eventually, we were able to comprehend the major aspects of our lives and there was there was nothing for the basic power to accomplish. In this way, it was able to be separated from rational reasoning. It is possible to add the fact that no one has been able to prove the existence of an essential power - it is completely inaccessible to science.

It is true it is, the rejection of the scientific method and superstition of the past has become an "elective prescription" of today. There are a few supposed "CAM" modalities that depend on vitalism, such as Reiki. Reiki actually is basically the same as therapeutic contact, which is a second method of regaining vitality that was popular among medical professionals however, despite the fact that it continues using it, it's significantly less popular after a an elderly woman of over a year (Emily

Rosa) carried out a remarkable test to show that it was just self-deceit. Reiki was able to fill in the gap.

The research on Reiki and the healing of vitality after all is said and completed, is reminiscent of a variety of modalities that are comparable - that have a very low credibility and logical validity that aren't given the attention they deserve in the field of restorative research. The study is of generally low-quality small, poorly controlled studies which appear to validate Reiki instead of determining if it is actually effective. The most recently widely-used examination, for instance examines the tension levels and self-proclaimed prosperity in malignant growth patients. The study also finds that patients feel more relaxed in the presence of the caring attention of an attendant. The exam is not controlled, and is has a questionable value. It is important to consider this type of investigation as a complete effort that is futile and ineffective since the outcome was not in doubt.

The current research does not allow any conclusions regarding the efficacy or effectiveness of healing the body's vitality. The future research should adhere to current norms of research regarding the efficacy and effectiveness of treatments as well as the stupendous character of the potential outcomes the cross-disciplinary philosophy could be necessary. In order to broaden the scope of preclinical investigations psychosocial processes, they should be examined and studied and not dismissed as fake treatments.

The current tests are of such poor quality that it is difficult to make any useful conclusion from it. If I differ to the contrary, and be that as it may, but this fundamentally means that we need to conduct more research. The lack of trust in the use of supernatural energy that has never been proved to exist by scientific research suggests something else.

Furthermore, the final sentence is a bit odd, as it suggests the authors are trying to transform misleading effects into real ones. This is the typical practice of the eminent drug advocates, as it is obvious that the vast majority of the methods they endorse aren't any better than fake treatments (which implies they're not effective).

Reiki is currently unambiguously within that group. It was released at the same time to the survey (and consequently not included from an audit) is a carefully planned investigation of Reiki in which Reiki was distinguished from false treatment Reiki (somebody who has not been trained for Reiki simply makes a small effort) in contrast to regular examination (no mediator). Like you would expect, both the authentic Reiki and the fake Reiki gatherings showed greater self-declared prosperity, more so than the non-intercession gathering however, they were not distinguished in comparison to one another. This means that Reiki wasn't more superior than false treatment. This means that Reiki does not work (at at all within the usual world of a scientifically-based prescription).

The creators wrap with:

The research shows that the proximity of an RN providing one-on-one assistance during chemotherapy could be effective in boosting solace and prosperity levels, irrespective of an effort to repair the vitality field.

I'm surprised that the creators weren't able to conclude "I can conclude that reiki doesn't work." This is oddconsidering that both treatment and fake treatment gatherings had the same effect on abstract results. When we use normal therapeutic mediations, we can conclude that the treatment does not work. Imagine a pharmaceutical company close:

The research shows the fact that taking a medication during chemotherapy could be beneficial in increasing the levels of comfort and happiness in combination with or without the use of a functional fix.

This is why taking pills is beneficial. There is no need to be concerned about whether dynamic fixing causes an impact on our bodies in particular. Reiki supporters have removed a section from the handbook for needle therapy. If real and fake needle therapy is superior to no treatment (they claim) and needle therapy is effective regardless of whether it's genuine or fake.

In a bid to ensure that patients will not receive fake therapies like Reiki research also suggests getting drugs that perform better than false treatment. For instance, back rub has been proven to boost the health of patients suffering from malignant growth, despite the illusion of. If the patient receives a back rub using compassion, compassion, patience as well as understanding and commitment the patient will benefit from the deceitful effect - much as Reiki persevering - however, in addition it is also possible to benefit from the specific effects of the treatment back rub provides and Reiki isn't able to provide.

This is an important aspect that I've been making over the years. There is no way to validate inadequate medications simply because they have false impressions. This is because legitimate medicines also have a similar effect, but also provide specific benefits since they actually perform.

I believe there are also a lot of possible harms from convincing patients that non-traditional treatments are necessary because of their ambiguous and misleading effects. This is a ploy that ignores self-government and educated consent and makes them vulnerable to possibly rely on ineffective "otherworldly" medicines for non-self-restricting diseases.

In the end when doctors or other social insurance specialists to recommend a treatment or amending practices to patients, they must prove that the practice is safe and efficient. Regarding security, there's been no specific negative effects of Reiki on any exploratory studies. This is logical given that no substance has been ingested or linked to the skin or the skin. Reiki contact isn't manipulative (and can be administered off the body in the event of need).

Is Reiki viable?

The question is what is Reiki practical? On the contrary, more precisely from an exploration standpoint what exactly is Reiki suitable for?

A Reiki specialist would answer the question with "Reiki is successful for reestablishing harmony, which can appear in various ways, contingent upon the ebb and flow need of the person." This isn't the kind of answer that appeals the therapeutic analysts who have a habit of diagnosing illnesses with specific medications instead of relying on medicines to improve health or restore harmony.

The purpose of restorative research as it is known is to answer a variety of questions. Although the standard drug has since recently incorporated an idea of homeostasis which is a fundamental level of equalization there's been no clear meaning to this notion that could be used to test the hypothesis that Reiki helps to improve equilibrium. Because of the ambiguity of the concept pressure and the differences in human bodies and the environments that they reside as well, what could the scientific method determine a person's parity?

What are the outcomes that have been considered?

The primary findings analyzed through Reiki research have relied on methods to treat anxiety, tension and stress, such as circulation strain, pulse, salivary cortisol as methods to combat burnout in the workplace and mind quality. More and more explicit measures are being used to evaluate the results of the recovery of strokes, depressive symptoms as well as other unending health ailments. Due to the relatively unpretentious and intricate character of Reiki practice the results of these tests may not be able to capture the actual knowledge of those who receive Reiki. Measures that connect happiness, peace of mind and stress reduction may be the most effective for showing the benefits that come from Reiki practice.

What are the various issues to be considered when researching Reiki?

Examining modalities, for example, Reiki raises different inquiries.

Quality of the randomized controlled preliminary tests

The controlled and randomized initial can be used to evaluate the impact of pharmaceutical products (albeit continuous improvements have shown that this type of demand is possible to control).

In any event, does the straightforwardness of the controlled, randomized study suitable for examining treatments that clearly trigger complex, multi-leveled, rapid and long-lasting reactions, for instance, as is the case by Reiki? Some experts think it's that it is not, and a discussion on how to best approach Reiki as well as other integrative therapies and healing practices has begun. The Frameworks hypothesis is increasingly recognized as providing a better method to focus the dangers of connecting in integrative therapies. The subjective approach could provide an additional basis for generating vital data. One of the most difficult variables in Reiki research is the ability to control the impact that human touches have on the body. Are Reiki recipients have better outcomes after receiving continuous contact from humans? Additionally, how can you create a fake treatment commonplace for a hands-on mending method? In 1999, the institutionalization of fake treatments was introduced into Reiki research, showing reviewers were unable to distinguish the character of fake treatments as well as Reiki experts. The development of an arm of fake treatment in Reiki research reinforces the investigation structure and tackles the perplexing issue in human-to-human touch. The inability to record the biofield. Another obstacle in Reiki investigation is inability of modern technology to document the existence of the biofield. This is significantly less to study its cosmetics, or track changes in it. Superconducting quantum-impedance devices (SQUIDs) measure extremely small attractive fields, and could be later useful to this study. The speed at which technological advancements are made could indicate that the needed technology is at the cutting edge of development. It is also possible it is possible that Reiki or biofields fall in the non-bioelectromagnetic zone. However, it's not necessary for scientists to document the presence of Reiki or the biofield to determine the impact on the human body. Reiki in the human body (headache treatment was used for many years before the science began to discover how it works). Although some effects of Reiki can be measured like a lowered circulation and pulse, numerous of the benefits normally described by repeated Reiki sessions, such as feelings of profound trust and improved confidence aren't measured. It is still essential to document these benefits in detail.

Patients who feel more deeply connected and simply rest in a state of mind about themselves could be people who are easier to treat and are more prepared to follow the treatment options. This is why

Reiki could be perceived to fundamentally, but in a tangent influence therapeutic outcomes by assisting patients to take their normal prescriptions and to draw more focus on their own requirements.

What is the current status of exploration?

As the debate about the best way to approach integrative therapies, like, Reiki is picking up momentum, exploration efforts have been and continue to be being created. Whatever the case, research into Reiki is just beginning.

Some other distributed studies have examined the effects of Reiki on the proportions of pressure hormones, pulse the insusceptible response as well as on reports of emotional distress of distress, anxiety and depression. The studies to date are typically small, and only one of every examination that is generally organized. However, information from a few of the more grounded tests bolster the capability of Reiki to alleviate anxiety and tenseness, and suggest its ability to speed up unwinding, alleviate the burdensome side effects and weaknesses and boost overall prosperity. It is the Cochrane Database of Systematic Reviews includes an assessment of the use of touch-based treatments (counting Reiki) for torment and a recommendation for the use of Reiki to treat mental issues.

Reiki is increasingly offered as an element of workplace wellness initiatives to reduce stress and increase capabilities in medical services and various businesses, as well as in health-related programs for students at colleges.

Chapter 8: History Of Reiki

REIKI is an ancient Tibetan form of healing. (pronounced Ray Key, it's an Japanese word that translates to universal energy or lifeforce energy).REIKI was discovered in the middle of the 19th century through Doctor. Mikao Usui.

Dr. Usui was the top of a Christian Faculty in Kyoto, in Japan. His students told him one day that they'd never had any idea of the methods for healing used for healing by Jesus Christ., they demanded the Dr. Usui in case he could perform this particular healing method for them. Unfortunately, they were not able to do it. Dr. Usui didn't have the details for the students of his, and as a result his resignation as the head of the Faculty and embarked on a quest to seek out the solutions.

He was in America to study and earned a higher education in Theology at Theology at the Faculty of Chicago. After that, he traveled to Japan to study the healing methods that were taught by Sutra and Buddha. Chinese Buddha and Sutra, before heading to Tibet where he studied Sanskrit (the ancient language of The Tibetan and India) Lotus Sutra. In this particular place, he found the answers he was looking for, the answers to the healing methods taught by Christ. He needed the power now.

He traveled to Japan and went to Japan and climbed Kuri Yama, the Holy Mountain of Kuri Yama in which he fasted , and was meditative for twenty days, in order to understand the essence of the Sanskrit method. He set up twenty one stones in front of him and each day that passed, the stone would be removed. While at the top of the mountain Dr.Usui read sutras, meditated, and sang. Dr.Usui was doing this for twenty-one days but nothing happened until the final day. The morning began but it was quiet and dim, he noticed a bright light moving toward him at a brisk speed. As it got closer, it got bigger on impact and grew in size him in the temple.

He observed a number of tiny bubbles of pink, lilac and the majority of the colors of rainbow. It was believed that Dr. Usui believed he'd died when a brilliant white light appeared before him. He was looking up and saw the well-known Sanskrit symbols in front of him, shining in Gold and he responded with a' Yes, I remember'. This was the beginning of the Usui method of REIKI.

After he was back to his reality, the sun released with the sky He was brimming with passion, he was alive, full of power and energy And even though he'd fasted for his Holy Mountain for twenty one days, he ran along the mountain. This was the beginning of magical moment.

In the rumble of his descent down the mountain and he stomped on the heel of the. He put it on the fingers of his and within a couple of minutes the bleeding stopped, and discomfort stopped. The next miracle was.

In the rush to climb the mountain, in the hurry to get on his mountain, Dr. Usui knocked the toe of his. He swaddled the hands of his near to the foot of his feet for just a few seconds and the bleeding and the pain went away. The next miracle was.

In the absence of food for twenty-one days, he became hungry, he stumbled across an Inn along the side of the road and bought the huge Japanese breakfast. The owner of the Inn advised him to not eat the food in such a large amount after fasting so long. However, the doctor. Usui managed to complete the meal without difficulty. It was the ultimate miraculous moment.

The daughter of the innkeeper's keeper was clearly struggling a lot of times with toothaches. Doctor. Usui placed the hands of his gentle on the face that was inflamed of her, and she began to feel better immediately. She rushed to her grandfather and made it clear that he was not a ordinary monk. It was her fourth miracle of the day.

Dr. Usui returned to his abbey in Kyoto to help the people of his abbey in Kyoto to treat the people from Beggar City and also the Slums. In his seven years of treating those in the shelter, he observed that the same people were coming into his care. He inquired about why they didn't move to a new life. They told him they should start begging because it was too difficult. Doctor. Usui was surprised by this, and realized that he had forgotten something important in the healings that were giving the beggars appreciation

The Dr. Chikiro Hayashi, one of Dr. Chikiro Hayashi. Usui's most trusted colleagues, developed into the new REIKI Grand Master within the course of the traditional. He was the owner of his personal Clinic of his in Tokyo from 1940 to the present. He treats unusual and serious cases. In the case of serious issues, REIKI is available round all hours of the day.

Around 1900, a lady called Hawayo Takata came into this world on the island of Hawaii Her parents her were Japanese and she was citizens of the United States. She was widowed, and had 2 children who were still young. Through 1935, the path that led her brought the way to REIKI. She was suffering from an illness of serious severity at the time and an inner voice urged her to seek treatment in Japan.

Mrs. Takata went to Japan in search of ways to heal. She was laying on an operating table every when a voice spoke to her and explained that there was absolutely no need to continue the procedure. The doctor asked her about different options for therapy and he also advised her to visit Doctor. Hayashi's REIKI Clinic. Thereafter, REIKI was put on to Ms. Takata every day by two providers. Within several monthsshe had returned in full health.

Hawayo Takata grew into a student of Dr. Hayashi for a year after when she returned in Hawaii with her two daughters. She was appointed as a Master in the presence of Dr. Hayashi as he visited Hawaii in 1938. She succeeded as Grand Master in 1941. She lived, was healed and also became qualified REIKI Masters. On December 11, in 1980, Hawayo Takata passed away and she was the first of twenty-two REIKI Masters throughout the USA and Canada.

Chapter 9: Reiki Energy Massage Treatment

Reiki is an acronym for two words: Rei as well as Ki. Rei refers to a large area, while Ki is a reference to streams of vitality or life. According to Reiki vitality healing, there are seven vitality centers, or known as chakras, on the spine of the body. A Reiki healer can accomplish this task by opening their crown chakra to general life force, and then direct or center the vitality of their hands to the patient. It is possible to perform this particular kind of healing in a specific area or even from an area of separation.

In recent times, many people have been looking for Reiki to heal, while they are undergoing various forms of medication. According to the firm instructors of Reiki healing, the physical, emotional and spiritual well-being is affected whenever a person's life-stream energy is affected or impeded in any way. Reiki is a safe and atypical mending option because it's non-intrusive and mostly uses the all-inclusive life force.

Reiki recuperation comes with a lot of medical benefits. For instance, it helps in loosening the body of the receiver which assists in releasing tension and anxiety. Once the body and brain are no longer full of tension, the safe framework becomes healthier and body becomes prepared to fight sickness by itself. Another benefit of Reiki that is being accounted for is the elimination of sleep deprivation as well as other slumber problems.

It is logical, knowing that when body, the psyche and soul are in a state of relaxation the rest is a regular occurrence. The reduction of hypertension is a recognized benefit of Reiki along with increased imperativeness and resistance. Another benefit of this treatment option that promotes otherworldly growth is the escalating of the body's vibration frequency.

In some manners, Reiki healing is similar to a back rubs, where the patient is lying on a table that is similar to the table used for back rubs, fully dressed. The air is also the form of a spa, from the delicate lighting to the music that is played softly and quietly.

The healing process begins with the recuperating doctor placing his hands on various areas of the patient's body. The procedure is carried out with a gentle touch and hands are usually put on the patient's body for a couple of minutes. Each healer has their specific strategies. Some healers are performing their hands freely according to the vitality flow of the patient.

Contrary to many believe, Reiki mending is not religious, however its effect is profound. The people who profit from this comprehensive treatment method, come from various religions and cultures. Even those who do not believe in Reiki recuperating, do benefit of it. This means that, to make it work, it is not a have to believe in it.

Chapter 10: The Definition Of Reiki:

Reiki is an Japanese word that is composed by two syllables: kanji (Japanese vowels):

REI - universal divine, love cosmic, vital;

K - energy, motion or vibration.

Combining these two words, we can comprehend the real meaning behind Reiki: Universal Energy, Spiritual Energy Vital Universal Force as well as energy of Unconditional Love, etc. Even though the word Reiki is Japanese it is a universal word. Reiki Energy is Universal.

Modern science has come to the realization that the Universe is composed of waves and vibrations. Reiki can be one. It is the vibration of Love and Harmony.

REIKI is an ancient Japanese natural technique of energy where the hands are employed to guide the energy to connect for it. Vital Energy of the Universe. The intention behind REIKI is to restore our energy, to ease us, lower stress levels and to enhance the quality of our lives by the growth of our personality and our physical, energetic emotional, mental, and spiritual equilibrium.

All living things have the capacity to recover their health naturally. Human bodies have all the resources needed to function, protect itself from harm and regenerate itself through its bodily processes, hormonal and immune system, and so on. Our ancestors were aware of all the rules of the Universe and live in the harmony of them. They understood and utilized the brain's intelligence as well as nature's laws and the information they gathered was transferred to the next generations. Humans sometimes act out in a way that is innate and ancient intelligence.

For example, we put our hands in the site that hurts because of a reflex that was inherited from our ancestral ancestors. Reiki is a proven method that helps us make use of our hands to create the vitality and harmony in our bodies through tapping into the universal Energy and (unconditional) love. All living things and humans are able to receive Reiki in its three types:

Reiki is the energy that powers the flow of life (natural life force),

Reiki as an activity that is spiritual (the spiritual power),

Reiki as an auto-healing technique (the strength of the body's physical).

Reiki works because it's energy that comes from the Heavens It is also known as Universal energy, and it radiates. Though it is a non-visible energy, people who are practicing Reiki may be able to see it.

Reiki Energy helps all living things to be in balance. Since the energy is of nature it assists in the evolution of life. Compare this with "artificial" energies (Roentgen, cobalt isotopes, etc.) that, if utilized excessively, can cause harm to living organisms. Human beings are the ultimate creation benefitting from individual consciousness , and is able to access more information and energies than all living things and is able to use these energies to improve its health. It is because of the illusions, materialism, upsets and fears that we show an tendency to overlook the benefits we have received through the Universe.

If we want to be channel for Reiki energy, Reiki energy, we must remove our limitations and open ourselves for Nature in general and to the Universe accepting our natural, unreservedly and provide us with the potential of Reiki. This is crucial to ensure that we are well-balanced and healthy throughout all areas of our lives. When we practice Reiki there is a possibility of feeling anxiety at first, but we will be able to observe the effects as we progress, and eventually we will be able to provide Reiki to those who are sick without hesitation or fear.

The student's observation is "I don't believe in auras or energies. How can I affect the energies?"

15-18 years ago, my answer on this issue was extremely basic, because the information I was able to access at the time was scarce. I would cling to words and try to explain it by citing a list of ideas that seemed to be logical from the perspective of the physics I was taught in the school curriculum: matter is created by atoms that contain an nucleus (protons and neutrons having positive charges) within which electrons move. So because we are talking about movement/gravitation/vibration; I concluded that because there is movement, there is energy.

In biology, we were taught that on a cellular level mitochondria convert the ingested nutrients into energy.

I also realized from physics that nothing goes away, everything transforms. If there is movement and transformation, there are ways through that these could be affected and synchronized.

Nowadays, we can access an abundance of information and research on the significance of energy and energy fields, consciousness, and divinity. The book serves a different purpose since I did not set out to write a science-based book on the subject. For those who are curious, skeptical or who are like me and aren't looking to make simple assertions and want to know more I will briefly explain the relationship with these methods of science. Then, you can independently go on to study if you want to do so.

The book is filled with references to how to reach an equilibrium state on all levels, and also less arguments from science, because Reiki helps to balance the communications between two cerebral hemispheres, and enhances emotional intelligence. You must read the book using your brain and your heart to fully comprehend its meaning.

Quantum mechanics as well as quantum physics provide an intriguing approach to describe the behaviour of matter at the subatomic and subatomic levels and help explain phenomena for which neither Newtonian Physics or the electromagnetism theory provide enough or all-encompassing information.

Classic Newtonian Physics is founded upon the study of things in everyday tests that are repeatedly validated as well as tested and verified thus gaining a deeper understanding of the physical behaviour. Biologically speaking , the body is thought of as an array of organs with each organ having distinct and clearly defined functions. The body functions as an "precise and exact Swiss watch" with everything operating in accordance with a perfectly pre-established process. But in reality, things are different in nature as well as within our body. The information and energy that cells transmit is not being recognized. The significance and the intelligence of cells, which form the foundation of the body and organs, are not understood.

As physicists began to study the subatomic level of Matter, Newtonian principles and concepts were inadequate. Quantum mechanics concepts began to be developed between 1926 and. The following are notable names of those who advanced these ideas to the incorporation of the concept that consciousness is a part of quantum Physics: Max Born, Erwin Schrodinger, Werner von Heisenberg (uncertainty principle, which defines the boundaries between concepts of classical Physics and the theories in quantum mechanics), Pascual Jordan, Wolfgang

Pauli, Niels Bohr (the Bohr-Bohm Theory), Paul Dirac, John von Neumann, Stephen Hawking, Nassim Haramein, Amit Goswami.

Quantum mechanics is founded on mathematical formalism, which describes physical phenomena with the help of space operators and vectors, and its measurements aren't based on determination. As an example, the particles don't follow well-defined orbits and are instead characterized by probabilities. Through time, several theories were proposed, pertaining to the method of measuring particles that are subatomic, since there are always uncertainties caused by probabilities. Niels Bohr wrote: "We can only know the probable position of a moving particle, therefore by extension, we can only know its probable destination; we can never know with absolute certainty where it will go."

The first major scission in quantum physics was created due to the conflict over Albert Einstein and Niels Bohr. Through the theories of relativity using the formula for relativity E = mc2. Albert Einstein surprised the scientific community of his day by showing that space and time are not distinct entities and are not solely connected but form an entire space-time continuum. The majority aspects of Einstein's contributions to physics relate to his theory of special relativity which incorporates electromagnetism, mechanics, and mechanics as well as to the general relativity theory which extends the concept of the general relativity of chaotic motion. Many publications on quantum physics claim the fact that Albert Einstein supported the idea that "the field is the sole governing agency of the particle." This is which has been confirmed by the outlooks, religions and oriental philosophies over many thousands of years: "spirit creates matter". In Einstein's work, we can mention his quantum theories of ideal gas monoatomic and, even though quantum theory was among the immediate outcomes of his research, Einstein was not a fan of the interpretations given to this theories through Niels Bohr as well as Werner Heisenberg.

Einstein was involved in heated discussions with the famous physicist Niels Bohr regarding the uncertainty principle, which would be a result of uncertainty and the probabilistic character of mathematical representations in quantum Physics. He wrote the following statement in an email addressed to Max Born, a physicist Max Born in 1962, in reference to Bohr's uncertainty principle: "I am convinced that God does not play dice". To Bohr, Bohr said: "Then stop telling God what to do with them." According to the theory of relativity (deterministic theory) dices appear uncertain, but by knowing the precise details of their motion it is possible to know how they'll fall.

Einstein passed away without acknowledging Bohr's quantum theory , but helped to develop the theory through his research.

Niels Bohr was a Danish scientist, developed the first quantum model structure of the atom (bearing his name) and also made important discoveries into the understanding of subatomic structure as well as quantum mechanics.

The neuropsychologist and physicist David Bohm introduced the holistic method that posits that the universe cannot be considered in terms of separate units and, as such the fragmented view was replaced by a unified one that incorporates observers (consciousness) with the physical world. The Universe all things are part of a vast continuous continuum. Bohm said that within the Universe everything is part of the whole but with its own unique specific characteristics. Bohm added that the Universe is just potential energy and energy.

The History of REIKI

There has been a lot written about the past of Reiki. There are two main versions, and their advocates tend to express their opinions in a way that is too loudly. Traditionally, information is passed through the mouth from Master to disciple, but not a lot of written information is provided. Because the history of Reiki is primarily built on communication of knowledge through oral channels, various versions have come to light.

I prefer an integrative approach to history by describing the documented history of Mikao Sensei and Reiki as well as that the Reiki "legend" from which I'll draw a few instances from the version that was presented by Ms. Takata and her changes that were attributed to her.

Even though healing techniques that involved the hands were practiced in a lot of the ancient civilizations, Reiki was developed through Mikao Usui Sensei, who was born in Japan in 1865 from the small village Taniai (today it is the town of Mijama). His dad, Uzaemon Cunetane, was an army commander. His mother was out of the Kavaai family. Usui learned about different practices of the oriental world and never went on to become a monk.

In the course of various life experiences Usui looked for and discovered the significance of life "Anshin Ritsumei" which means "Your spirit is at peace, and fully conscious of what you need to do with your lifeand being completely and unaffected." To attain this, he sat for 21 days between Feb and Mar 1922 at the top of Kurama which is about 12 km away from Kyoto and where he came across the resonance and connection to Reiki. Reiki vibration. In some of the books/histories it's stated that Usui initially started teaching the TEATE method, which means "healing with the hands". The name is derived from the work he was doing, not from his previous lessons. This method was prior to Reiki, which was the name of the United States University. RYOHO Method (meaning "The Reiki Usui healing method").

In the month of April 1922, Mikao Usui founded the USUI REIKI RYOHO Gakkai organization. In the beginning, to be able to practise Reiki followers were close to their master and Reiki was passed on through the Master's aura through the energy of followers. Initiations weren't performed in the manner they are nowadays. In fact, the Reiki symbols were later introduced by Mikao Usui to make Reiki practice more simple. However, today, there aren't all the symbols used in Gakkai.

I enjoy telling these story that come from my personal "legend" passed on by Ms. Takata. It's possible that they are not real however, because they were taught to me and became familiar with these stories, I love telling these stories. I accept responsibility and take responsibility for integrating these aspects into the past of Reiki which I teach at my classes:

a)When Mikao Usui made the decision to scale Mount Kurama he only took with the mountain 21 pebbles, one for every day. Every day, before sunrise, he would throw one pebble. The last day that he had only one pebble left, sitting in meditation, Mikao Usui was in a state of light and experienced a blissful state. After he regained his state of mind, he realized it was the moment desired result he'd been looking for since a long period of time. He also realized that he been able to enter the realm of Reiki energy. As he was walking down the mountain Mikao Usui sprained one of his legs . He immediately put his hand on the injured area and realized that his hands were extremely warm, the bleeding stopped , and healing began. This was for him the first evidence that the gift he obtained from the Universe was working.

At the base of the mountain, there was a shelter for pilgrims where he could eat. The lady who handed his food was suffering from a severe toothache. Usui requested permission to put his hands on her face, near her teeth. She agreed and after couple of minutes of keeping his hands close to her face, the discomfort diminished.

b)Following this "happenings" Mikao Usui settled down in Tokyo and established the retreat, where he offered treatment to individuals using Reiki. Mikao Usui decided to introduce the five Reiki principles to everyone who are practicing Reiki.

We are back to the actual story. In September 1923 following the earthquake that struck Japan, Usui and his disciples were helping victims. This is the way Usui and Reiki were recognized. The officers of the Japanese navy were informed concerning Reiki as well as Usui and asked Usui to instruct them on Reiki. A few navy officers were trained up to the Shinpiden level. Usui died on the 9th day of March 1926. His method was passed down by around 2000 people who practiced Reiki and the 21 disciples of Reiki Shinpiden. Twelve of 21 Shinpinden disciples are well-known to us.

In 1927, Gakkai creates Mikao Usui's monument to his funeral in Tokyo in the Saiho-ji Temple. Gakkai is the sole organization that has the authority to construct monuments or memorial plaques in honor of Usui. Gakkai continues to operate until today. Gakkai is an organization that has restricted access and only 500 members.

Usui Reiki Ryoho which is currently being referred to as Dento Reiki is only practiced in Japan The Reiki routes outside Japan are known as Western/Occidental Reiki.

Chujiro Hayashi, who was a ex- Navy official and military physician, as well as graduated from the Naval Japanese Academy came in contact with Reiki through Admiral Taketomi Usui's mentor. In 1925 Hayashi met Mikao Usui. A few versions of the story of Reiki claim that Usui demanded Hayashi to conduct some study about Reiki and to further develop the techniques for Reiki along with Reiki. Reiki practice. Following the death of Usui, Hayashi quit Gakkai and founded Hayashi Reiki Kenkyukai Institute. Hayashi Reiki Kenkyukai Institute, where he continued to conduct research.

Mrs. Takata was talking about the clinic established in the year 2000 by C. Hayashi where Reiki practitioners worked together in a group as volunteers for one year, providing treatment to patients at the clinic. It was a mandatory training required to attain the higher levels of Reiki (Okuden). Hawayo Takata was admitted to the clinic as an individual patient in the year 1935.

Chujiro Hayashi departed this world on May 11, 1940.

Hawayo Takata was born of Japanese origin. She was born on 24th December, 1900, at the shores of Kauai on the island of Kauai in Hawaii. She was widowed in her early years. Due to her health issues, she moved to Hawaii and headed to Tokyo to undergo surgery. She spoke with her doctor if there were other alternatives to surgery. He suggested the Hayashi clinic, where the patient. Takata got well within several months. After seeing the benefits of this technique , Ms. Takata wanted to learn Reiki and in 1973, she was awarded the level II and returned to Hawaii where she set up an Reiki clinic.

Chujiro Hayashi came to visit the woman in 1938, in Hawaii. He spent six months with her and admiring the results she obtained, he gave her the status of Reiki teacher on 21st of February , 1938.

The Ms. Takata is considered to be the Founder of Occidental Reiki. It was thanks to her, it gained recognition throughout the USA. It was during difficult historical times during which Japan along with the USA were at war and everything with Japanese origin was seen as suspect. After the attacks of December 1941 at Pearl Harbor the anti-Japanese sentiment among Americans increased. This is why it's normal to understand why Mrs. Takata "adapted" Reiki to fit better with the western way of life, adding aspects of Christianity into Reiki and abstaining from certain practices.

She began her Reiki courses by introducing the concept to the power of the Universe that she described as an infinite energy force that descends from the Creator/Source which surrounds us. She referred to this method as USUI SHIKI the RYOHO (meaning that it was the "Usui-style healing method "). Due to the limitations at the time, Ms. Takata modified a few aspects of Reiki techniques that were taught by Usui and Hayashi and to learn specific Reiki exercises, she earned an advanced diploma in massage.

Following the bombing by Japan in 1945 by USA in 1945, Ms. Takata no longer had relations with Japan. Hawayo Takata taught Reiki training for over forty years across Canada and the USA as well as Canada and in her last years of training, she taught 22 Reiki Masters.

The title Master was given to masters in Japan just to the people who have achieved the state of illumination. In contrast, Takata started using this title in the year 1970, when she began offering an initiation for the level of Reiki teacheror instructor. We must therefore clarify that the term "Reiki Master" in the West does not mean that a Reiki master in the West is not always an individual who has achieved illumination.

Madame. Takata left this world aged 80 she passed away on the 25th day of December, 1980. I have the greatest respect for Ms. Takata who was brave enough to advocate and practice Reiki in a difficult time in the history of humanity.

There are many different interpretations within the USA as well as in Japan concerning the process of Reiki following Ms. Takata's demise. But, Reiki, if it really is Reiki is similarly, equally within the west, East and in Japan.

Chapter 11: The Reiki Healing Tool

Physical Reiki improves the body's inherent capacity to heal it self. It helps rid the body of poisons and toxins, and helps to balance and harmonize the body, promoting wholeness and overall well-being. It also aids the body be aware of its basic and most essential need, like proper nutrition, exercise and sleep routines.

Emotional Reiki directly affects the emotional energy. It urges them to analyze the emotional reactions they have to people or situations, and also encourages positive emotions such as happiness, affection, love as well as trust, happiness, kindness, and trust. It also helps transform emotional energy into creative energy.

Mental Reiki alters the way one thinks and helps them let the negative thoughts that plague them. It also helps to promote positivity and peace. This leads to a state that is deep relaxation. Reiki uses your energy fields to increase the ability to sense. It enhances the person's consciousness and self-awareness, enabling them to attain their personal goals and goals.

Spiritual Reiki can affect the soul and the spirit. It affects the entire energy body, and assists individuals to be more accepting and loving of their own self. It also promotes more tolerance towards humanity, encouraging people to accept them just as they are, despite their various spiritual paths. It promotes compassion, love acceptance, tolerance, and helps one to be on the path of being in touch to the Divine.

No matter how we see it, the most evident is that you must take on the responsibility of your own well-being and health. Take part in your own self-healing. Reiki isn't a magic cure-all method, even though it can be extremely beneficial in helping you to achieve optimal health. It assists in removing discomfort and pain however, it is a commitment to accept attitudinal and lifestyle changes so that healing is total and permanent.

In order to practice Reiki it is essential to take the responsibility for your well-being. You must be able and able to feel the effects of the body's energy being stimulated. You should be able to gain a greater knowledge of what your body requires and give your body the respect it deserves with love and respect.

Thus, if you are using Reiki daily but persist following habits and practices that aren't healthy for your emotional, spiritual physical and mental health Your body will go responding negatively. That's why Reiki isn't unstoppable. It is not able to be effective until you are consciously allowing it to.

This is the thing that Reiki First Degree is all about the power of using Reiki on yourself to heal yourself. Reiki eliminates blockages within your energy system, gradually traversing the layers of energy stagnation that are most likely to be caused by negative thoughts or unhealthy habits that will frequently come to mind as thoughts when you start Reiki. It is a "letting go" process is extremely important.

When the memories are revealed and the memories are triggered, you have the chance to heal and gain from the experiences. It may take months, weeks or even years, but you'll find yourself more vibrant, energetic and fulfilled as the process progresses.

Experiencing Reiki Healing

Typically, the client is completely clothed on a massage table, and the Reiki practitioner rests his/her hands close to the body of the client. It is vital to keep in mind that Reiki is a divine power, and since it operates holistically, it may not be able to operate exactly the place where the practitioner has placed his or her hand. The energy can address the root cause of pain in the body regardless of what the patient isn't conscious of. A good example would be, for instance when one suffers from an anxiety-related headache the life force or ki energy won't just address the pain of a headache but also proceed to treat the mental state of the patient that can be causing the headache.

The Reiki master positions his or her hands in various hand positions for between 2 and 10 minutes, based on the length of time required for each hand position. The whole treatment is likely to last from 45 minutes to one hour. Based on the condition of the patient and needs, they may need to repeat the sessions bi-weekly or, if they discover that they have completely healed after this one session, or in no way.

Different people experience various Reiki experiences. Many people experience an intense calm. There is also a glowing radiance or energy. Others experience visions, or an experience of being out of body. Sometimes when the Reiki Practitioner detects obstructions in the chakras clients may experience initially a feeling of heavyness, followed by an exhalation and then an energy flow.

Chapter 12: Reiki And Your Chakra

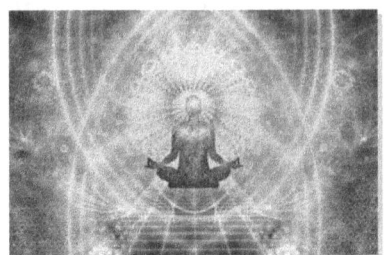

All around us there is energy that changes constantly. Our bodies absorb this energy in the form of sponges and then it gets absorption through your chakras.

The awareness of the chakras within the body of a person has been present from before the dawn of the modern age and they play an essential part in yoga.

In Sanskrit the word "chakra" literally refers to "wheel of light" and that's why chakras ought to be viewed as a present, particularly for those who can perceive them. If someone is able to see them they appear to be spinning light wheels. Each chakra appears to be a distinct color in the spectrum of the rainbow.

Every chakra lies with the spine and make up the backbone which connects the mind, body and the spirit. This network comprises a variety of smaller energy centers within the body. They are usually associated to Acupuncture points.

When you are having an Reiki session, hands are placed on the principal chakras and the secondary chakras. These tend to be discolored and dysfunctional or completely shut off because of issues with one's body, mind or body. It is essential to keep these channels open as if there is an interruption in the energy flow, it can result in illness.

When Usui created his version of Reiki The Japanese culture didn't think of the energy of the body as chakras. Instead, they focussed more on the hara that is the area between the navel and the pubic bone. This is the center of body's gravity. Also, there is an tanden that is located on the middle of the chest, just above the eyebrow.

However, the knowledge of chakras in the past brought value to Reiki that was practised throughout the globe. In the present, Reiki is practiced everywhere and is based on the significance of chakras.

The purpose of Reiki treatments is to assist in clearing chakra blockages as well as restore the flow of the life energy.

Energy flows into and out of the aura via the chakras. This is a shining energy that surrounds everyone. The aura is comprised by seven distinct layers each is responsible for the different aspects of our lives. The chakras of the major chakras form an elongated cone that surrounds the center of our spine that runs through each layer in our aura.

Within the physical body, every major chakra is connected to an endocrine gland which helps to regulate the balance of hormones as well as a significant nerve plexus.

At the base of the spine it is where the chakra of root. between the genitals, and the naval are the sacral chakra. above it is the solar plexus chakra. In the center of your chest lies the heart chakra. between your neck, there is the throat chakra. below the brow is a third eye chakra, and above the head is the crown chakra.

There are more than 100 minor chakras that are present in the body that are involved in Reiki.

Balancing Chakras

If your chakras are in balance you'll feel more relaxed. You might be able to tell that your chakras aren't in balance when you start to feel sick. Here are some methods that you can apply to balance your chakras using Reiki.

Put your one finger on the chakra of crown, and another on your root chakra.

Moving each hand further away from the body that is sensing chakra energy.

If you experience less energy around one chakra, then you could place both hands on the chakra by using Reiki to help bring the chakra back to its normal position.

Continue to use Reiki till you experience the exact sensation sensation with both hands. It should be a feeling of balance and balance to feel confident to move on to your next chakra.

Your next appointment will begin by laying your hands on your third eye chakra , as well as the sacral chakra.

Repeat the process until your chakras are in balance.

Continue to move through the chakras until you are done balancing all chakras.

You must believe in your own intuition during this process , and ensure that you leave your patient calm and balanced. If you are doing the regular chakra balance, people might start to get insights into the issues that lie in the deep layer of their chakras. It is important to determine whether Reiki will suffice to take care of the impurities, or if additional therapies are required to balance the patient.

Chapter 13: The Third Chakra

The chakra of the third is often referred to as the fire chakra, or in Sanskrit the manipura. It is associated with ego and power, and is usually the predominant chakra for people with imbalanced chakras. The fire chakra is situated in the solar plexus. This is the reason why, if you are feeling anxious, scared and insecure, or even in love, you may feel feelings of butterflies or a heavy feeling near or even beneath the solar plexus. The chakra of fire is restricted by the emotion of shame.

Third chakra regulates the ability of us to form close connections with people and places that we consider essential. For instance that satisfaction and joy that you feel when you get at home after having been away for many years is tempered through the chakra of fire. It's surprising that the third chakra is responsible of balancing ego and power in the same way that it determines how we see and behave when we interact with others. Do you remember the expression "power partner"? There's a reason behind why the term is frequently associated with intimate relationships as well as the existence of power battles among the couples in the relationship.

The fire chakra is opened.

The importance of the fire chakra lies in since, after you've learned to let away guilt and fear it is important to realize that you are able to accomplish what you wish to and be the person you wish to be. The fire chakra is a way to teach people that the true power lies in being able to leverage authority and influence to promote interests, aid others and contribute to the world. To activate your chakra's third, you must follow the steps below for a quick and easy way to do it.

Step 1: Search for the location that offers direct access to warm. It is best to choose a place that is calm and bright. You could also relax next to the fireplace.

Step 2. Preparing your body as well as your mind for the sensation that will open the chakra of your third. Think about the sensation of connecting to your first and second chakras. Invoke the energy of the earth and the water that is in the ground or within the air surrounding you. Be aware that all the elements, as well as the chakras you have connected.

Step 3. Relax or sit comfortably in the front of the fireplace or in the sun. Some even lay on the ground or on the floor in order for the complete force of the warmth on their bodies. Put your hands upon your solar plexus and breathe in a steady and consistent way.

Step 4: Think about the people, things locations, and events which have created a sense of power. Consider how you used influence and power at the time you were in control and why you were able to gain them at all.

5. Now, think about the actions you've done with shame. Consider the way you felt. Did you feel helpless? Do you feel like you are powerless? Do you ever feel like giving up? Did you ever feel ashamed of your shortcomings?

Step 6: Remember that third chakra can teach people to manage power, and to use it to benefit others, and to assist in helping oneself and others to grow. Consider the times when you were in control and had influence and how it affected your relationships and your perceptions. Consider the times when you were embarrassed and felt embarrassed about you or your situation. Consider all of these issues and let them slowly go. Imagine the fire chakra's powerful power consuming your disappointments and shame. Visualize the fiery chakra sustaining your compassion and achieving accomplishment.

Step 7 Take a deep breath and breathe slowly. Each time you breathe reflect on your shortcomings. Each time you exhale remind yourself that each person has each of their own flaws and that, despite your imperfections and shame, you should learn to love yourself as you are. Recognize that it's through loving your entire self that you will grow into the true power of balance.

The fire chakra can be strengthened by connecting or wearing to objects with yellow in their color. The third chakra is recharged by eating certain foods like cereal, pasta bread, flax seeds, bread and yogurt.

Chapter 14: The Difference Between Reiki And Angelic Reiki

There are many differences between Reiki methods that are practiced in the world as well as Angelic Reiki.

It's generally accepted that the method of healing referred to as Reiki is the primary method of healing which was utilized in Atlantis. It's generally accepted that the culture of Atlantis was more advanced in its consciousness when it came to connecting with Divine Wisdom, more so than what we have today.

They used vibrational symbols to attain God's power. Using them within a closed system as the body, could bring balance and harmony. This is how healing happens.

The Differences

The healing mechanism at the time of Atlantis was discovered by Dr. Usui in the early 1880s because humans are at the opposite end of the 26,000-year cycle of the solar system. This is the time when Atlantis was destroyed.

The healing system that Dr. Usui discovered was rigorously protected by the tradition of authenticity of transmitting the spells Dr. Usui utilized.

The humanity's spiritual perception in the 1880s was awed by the idea the fact that humanity was part of an larger system known as"the Solar System. What this means is that intellectual/spiritual human race at that time could only comprehend themselves to be part of the Solar System. The symbols Dr. Usui employed were made available to use with the frequency of the human race at the time that was solar consciousness.

In the years since 1880, humans have expanded its consciousness at an exponential rate. Following World War 2, a increase in consciousness allowed humans to increase their consciousness to accept the notion that we're a solar system within the galaxy of lots different solar system. This could be referred to as galactic consciousness. The majority of Reiki methods that have been developed in the past few years have been based on the existing Reiki symbols and have made these symbols are correlated with Heart chakra. In the Harmonic Convergence of 1987 another increase in consciousness has occurred that allows these Reiki symbols be distributed with higher frequencies than the heart chakra.

When Angelic Reiki was first conducted in 2003, the attunements of the symbols took place in the throat chakra. In recent times, for this first time ever since Atlantian times, the healing symbolism of Atlantis are being utilized at all seven levels of form and Divine Form.

The practice of Angelic Reiki all of the symbols employed are used to complete the seven levels of form and Divine Form.

Since the beginning of time, and with the entire mysteries of the school, experiences in the mind were revealed by the master to the student by way of initiation.

Prior to initiations, there is often an initiation. Movement. through which the pupil must prove through via physical testing, their capability to be eligible for the

The practice was somewhat reduced by the New-Age

Initiation is an energetic awakening of the Masters consciousness that has been infused into pupils' consciousness. It's a merging, an over-lighting of one consciousness with another to increase the frequency and consciousness of that consciousness to the shining illumination that is the master.

Some of the attunements that are offered today through the Reiki system aren't of the highest quality. The person receiving this attunement may become influenced by a conscious which is still struggling with emotional issues, ego-related issues and personal connections.

The Angelic Reiki system has always been associated with a method of healing that, uses symbols that communicate with the Divine Archetypal energies that attune the seven human bodies to their divine original frequency.

In order to ensure that these symbols can be transmitted to pupils in their purest form and purity, they aren't given as an act of initiation by the teacher. This teacher creates the space that is a vortex of energy and the Angelic Kingdom is able to manifest their energy around every pupil and secures the symbol into the chakras that are appropriate.

The symbols are then delivered at a divine frequency, and consequently, they affect the mind of every pupil at the moment they're handed.

In this set of rules, it is the customary initiations 1 to 4. In addition there are two other rituals that are exclusively angelic.

The angelic kingdom was created as a result of the earlier evolution of the universe. It is therefore an enormous difference between the frequency of an Angel and that of a human who has been incarnated.

The Archangel Metatron took a firm belief that the induction of the Angelic Vibration is an integral part of the system.

I've learned that during these initiations, the atomic spin of every molecule within the body of the pupil receiving the attunement speeded up. This allows to enhance the power of the student more precisely synchronize with the energy of angels that are their constant companions in the wake of the initiation.

Chapter 15: Life With Three Eyes

The experience of having the Third Eye is quite different from living with only two eyes - the "standard issue" two. In this last chapter, we'll look at some of the changes and the new experience and feelings that you'll begin to experience in your daily life.

An Eye in the Back of Your Head?

You might have heard the phrase "they must have eyes in the back of their head" and when you've the Third Eye you could be able to view and experience your world from a different way. These abilities are usually the first to be developed as the complicated connection between our subconscious and conscious mind gets more in tune. Our subconscious is the storehouse of our experiences and many believe that it is the same in this and past ones. Once you've opened Your Third Eye you have far more access to this part of you and will soon be able to see patterns in your life as well as in the world around you. You'll become more adept at identifying the most likely outcomes of events. As time passes, this will develop into the truly "clairvoyant" abilities - the ability to see so clearly , it appears - or could be that you are able to predict the future.

Meet The Ancestors

While the Third Eye heals and develops there is a high possibility that your connection to the world of spirit, and your ability to communicate with the realm of spirit will be enhanced drastically. There are guides for all of us and we all are affected by the spirit world constantly. The most common manifestation of this is in people's lives as finding themselves in the correct spot at the right time or even noticing "uncanny" coincidences, which cause them to make an important choice. With a healthy, active and functioning Third Eye it will be more multi-directional and you might be able to sense spirits speaking directly to you. It is usually evident in the beginning, as you start to notice relatives or friends who have died. As time passes, this feeling will grow to include people who gather with other people as well as completely strangers.

Strange Vibrations

A lot of people experience these symptoms in the initial stages of decalcifying the Pineal Gland which opens their third Eye. The most frequent symptoms are a strong tingling in the region at the middle of the forehead, which is where it is believed that the Third Eye is usually depicted. Some people experience the sensation of a gentle tickling like being brushed by feathers. Others, however, feel it is one of constant pressing or a touch. In a small percentage of cases headaches , or migraines may be experienced. Although it is uncommon, they do occur on occasion. Headaches are usually gone within a few days, and usually less intense over the course of. The symptoms are documented widely and are not a cause for worry however they are simply a normal aspect in the course of. The tingling or a touch sensation is usually gone within a couple of weeks or, at the very least, become so commonplace that it's not noticed. A few people experience periods of insight, mediumship or clairvoyance, they feel or feel the same sensation. A lot of people with an active Third Eye take this to indicate that they need to make use of the skills (clairvoyance medium-ship, clairvoyance or even spirit contact) in the event that the feeling returns.

Alive and Dead

Death isn't an end, it's just it is a natural element of our spiritual journey. It is a necessary aspect in the process of opening Your Third Eye that you'll begin to having greater contact with the spirit world. In the initial days after the opening of your

Third Eye the contact will often take the shape of dreams. Friends or relatives who have disappeared could be present in the dreams of your more vivid ways than they did previously. Conversations with them may appear much more "real" in dreams and it's not a random occurrence! Be attentive to what they are saying and make sure you consider any advice they provide. Although spirits of all sorts offer a wider view of our personal worlds and the world around us, don't believe that you need to take their advice! Certain, the spirits you find you close to are educated, but you must take the time to learn (or be reminded) to make decisions based on your own brain and initiative and not trust advice from the realm of spirit.

The possibility of encountering spirits in dreams is common during the initial stage of the development of your Third Eye however, encountering them in the world of the living is not uncommon and increasing likely as you improve your abilities. Due to Hollywood our perception about "ghosts" is largely negative and could make you worry about your safety. However, the reality is that this perception is false; you're more likely to suffer injury from the physical side of a person, in the actual reality, then from any spiritual connections you create. The physical realm isn't the normal realm of spirit and it's all yours! Keep the idea in your mind you must be aware that you are able to make an effort to get unwanted, unpleasant or unhelpful spirits to go away. They will have no choice but to follow your instructions and your motive is crucial in this instance. Be sure to be clear in your words and use the words you say to spirits of any kinds. This applies to the people we live with too!

Heightened Sensitivity

This is often a neglected problem for those who are working on their new abilities. If you have a healthy, active Third Eye, you'll quickly be more observant and open to the feelings of people who are around you. This includes complete strangers when you walk by them on the streets. They are powerful. they can be good but they can also be a disaster. Being open to them could cause you to feel tired and exhausted. You'll notice that you're not willing to be around people who display negative emotions, and your feeling of empathy will grow rapidly as you look into the Third Eye. It is important to distinguish empathy with sympathy. You'll be able to feel how the person you're feeling as if they were feeling the same way.

When you begin the first steps to work with your Third Eye the best advice is to avoid people or situations where you are subject towards negative thoughts. They make you feel tired and make it difficult to fully utilize the Third Eye or reap the benefits of it. But, as you grow more comfortable with life using three eyes, you should consider the advantages the new "powers" can offer others. A significant aspect of spiritual development is how people interact in the environment around us, and especially, the manner how our actions towards other people are carried out. Utilizing those "powers" or abilities to profit only you can result in you becoming smaller, narrow-minded, and self-centered, which will end up destroying those abilities! Develop the strength to make use of your empathy to assist, improve and benefit the people surrounding you. Remember to take time to yourself. Walk through the mountains and woods by yourself, take a bath, meditate and think about daydreaming. Whatever "re-charges" your batteries, ensure that you set aside enough time for it like anything else. This will ensure you are equipped with the energy to apply your skills to the maximum effect.

Getting, or Staying, Physical

A lot of people have ignored their Third Eye for so long that opening it could be an quite an experience. It could become, at times like an obsession, but keep in mind that even though it's extremely crucial to your spiritual growth it is far from being the pure spirit. There are real, urgent physical requirements in our lives These are simple and consist of being fit and healthy as well as eating right and having fun. These things should be considered the cornerstones of your lifestyle. If you have an open Third Eye it is likely to discover that you're actually eager to eat well and live healthy You'll feel that way! Make sure you balance your emotional, physical and spiritual needs in your life, and set aside space for each of these.

New Friends and Old

As you progress in your spiritual development you may discover that certain people in your life do not meet your needs any more. Don't worry about it We all grow at times. As your spiritual and psychic development progresses, you'll look for new avenues for learning and growth. These can also bring new people to your life. Don't be unwilling to shed the past and look towards the future in all aspects within your personal life. It's not a reason to let friends or acquaintances go without a hitch You may share strong bonds with a lot of them, and they could influence your life in ways you've yet to uncover. If, however, some connections have been lost in your journey, you must accept that it's an inevitable part.

Patience, Patience, Patience

Be patient as you wait for to see the third Eye. The instructions and steps included in this book will assist to make the process more real and feasible, however it might take longer as compared to other people. If you already have greater spiritual awareness or natural clairvoyance, the process could be swift for days, weeks, or even a few months. Some people may be more prolonged, with advancement and delays along the way. Keep in mind to be persistent and patient as you might have to make a number of changes to your life as you grow and some may require some time and effort. The more times you test more, the better chances of success. Don't be tempted to be discouraged by small failures. Instead, get up and try again. It will happen!

Chapter 16: The Five Phases Of The Chi Cycle

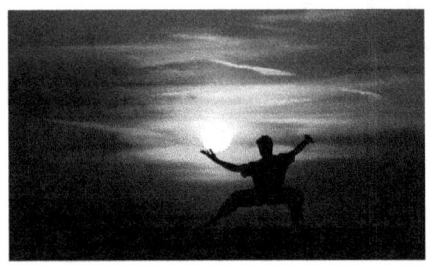

Matter, along with its condensed Chi and condensed Chi, is controlled through the Cosmic Chi and being the influence controlled through the Celestial Chi feeding itself with Telluric Chi results in life. These transformations and influences are exhibited in a polar Universe (positive-negative) that is manifested through the dissociation from Yin as well as Yang.

In the universe of this it is believed that everything exists in a constant fluctuation of Yin as well as Yang. The various states in which Chi moves between Yin into Yang as well as vice versa and the rules that govern this transition were outlined through the Taoists in the Five Phases of the Chi Cycle.

Chi exhibits specific characteristics throughout its journey through the phases. The phases are named symbolically by the natural elements in which these traits are clearly visible. They are"the Phase of Fire, Earth Metal, Water and Wood. These are the traits that Chi is able to adopt at each stage of its Yin-Yang transition.

The Five Phases of the Chi Cycle explain the dynamic nature of each cyclic motion throughout the universe. as we've already observed in the definition of terms like Yin and Yang the whole universe is a cycle and everything is subject to the laws of physics.

As described as part of The Five Phases.

This cycle of continuous repetition occurs throughout every living being and aspect of the universe as all things are subject to the Yin-Yang duality, and nothing is static. The creation and destruction of stars, as well as the life cycle of each living being as well as the various biological processes that take place inside living creatures. Every aspect is affected by this cycle.

In the Fire Phase, Chi is hot and increasing, reaching the highest manifestation of Yang. This is energy which transcends matter and expands outwards. It's the heat that is the immaterial, and the explosion. The ultimate of the transformation. It's summer, the endless of noon and the youth.

In the Earth phase, Chi is more passive, temperate , and binder. The Earth phase accepts the free energy and inert matter and combines them to create the new forms of Chi. It is at the heart in Chi Cycle. Chi Cycle, to which it returns at the end of every phase and then it goes on to following cycle. It is the shape and the end result, the fruit, as well as the raw material for the next cycle. Agglutinate, amalgam, digest, equate. It's harvest time halfway maturity, the start in the evening.

In the Metal Phase, Chi is contractive, delimiter, differentiator, and selective. Chi is a delimiter, differentiator and selective Yang that was warmed up during the Earth Phase now begins to slide toward the Yin aspect. Chi of Metal Chi of Metal tends to condense and accumulate, thereby absorbing the energy of matter. It is the Chi of Metal encourages the matter of energy, fills it up with Chi from life and creates pressure inside to stay outside the external world. It's condensation and internalization. It's autumn and the time of entry into the middle ages, and in the afternoon.

* In the Water phase, Chi descends and becomes paralyzeduntil it reaches the highest manifestation of Yin This is called materialization. The change and movement occur here until they reach their lowest expression. Energy is infused into the subject and is blessed with a

stable structure. The structure's validity is determined and the unnecessary is eliminated and destroyed. Chi remains imbued in matter. It reigns supreme in the immobility. The dance has been frozen however Chi continues to move forward in its journey of transformation. The transforming power that is Yang is stored in material and released when the conditions are right. The Yin waits for the appropriate time to release the energy it that it received. It's the seed. be patient for it. It's cold and wintery and old age, dark.

* In the Wood phase, Chi expands and mobilizes. Wood Chi is the energy that regulates the matter. "Yin holds Yang. Yang dominates the Yin" according to what the old saying goes. The Chi that is retained is argued, being influenced, mobilized from outside, and then dragging the subject matter back with the power of mobility and mover begins to adjust to the new environment, expand and life. The Chi

is the Yang which gives energy to Yin and warming it. It's growth, movement and expansion, ad-hocation. It's springtime, childhood, and the first day of the week.

Any being, whether it is either inanimate or animate and manifests in nature is made up of many different Chis, which have an yin or yang character, that react to a particular phase or other that comprise the Chi Cycle. Each of these influences puts the individual with the ability to be aware of its individual characteristics and the harmonious interaction between all of these forces permits that the being to remain for a period of duration. The discord between all of these forces that form the persona is due to the deterioration of the misno or development to a different state since everything in nature is prone to search for a place that is in balance.

The harmony between yin, Yang and the chi, which corresponds to the various stages that comprise the Chi Cycle, in addition to other concepts that are closer to the Western concept of the ratio of matter-energy and liquid heat and the matter-energy ratio, form the basis of understanding illness and health in the context that is a part of Chinese culture.

We know that the chi within each phase has certain specific features, however, the distinct types of chi do not exist on its own, but are interconnected with the chi from the other cycles that are accompanied by the constant motion. The interactions between Chi of various natures are studied in two different types of chi: the food or growth cycle, and controlling cycles.

Within the Growth Cycle, the Chi of each phase feeds into or powers the following phase. It is usually stated as "the mother feeds the child" The Water Phase is the one that feeds the Wood Phase The Fire Phase feeds the Wood Phase Fire Phase and so on.

In contrast in the Control Cycle it is usually said "that "the counselor moderates the emperor" The Chi from the Water Phase is controlled by those of the Fire Phase which is composed is made of metal, and so on.

The manifestations and beings of this universe will reveal the predominantity of certain types of manifestation of Chi. The connections between the various kinds of Chi will assist us to discover the interrelations between different beings as well as the connections that exist between the inner vital processes of every living thing.

Think about the following scenario the following scenario: The president who is newly elected to an organization, roughly forty-years old (land) which displacing and sets its own standards against those established by the previous President, currently an elder (water) in pursuit of his goals with the energy of younger workers (fire). So, fire feeds the earth which then is the one who controls the water. If the president of the past was concerned that his successor was abusing his authority, he could exercise an authority that he could directly exercise over employees. Thus, water could be able to control the fire, while restoring the balance of power by cutting off support for the property.

The Macrocosm and the Microcosm

In the universe beyond (macrocosm), Yin and Yang are manifested during the main climatic phases of winter and summer. The transition from one to the next is made through various stations that correspond to the five phases of Energy that are: The winter season (maximum Yin, predominance of Water Chi), Spring (predominance of Wood Chi), Summer (Fire Chi) and the late summer harvest and the intermediate months (Earth Chi) as well as Autumn (Metal Chi) and then we begin a new cycle.

Another macrocosmic cycle that involves Yin as well as Yang interactions is known as the cycle of day and night. In this manner it is the case that the Chi is transformed from and Yin to the highest Yang and back to Yin through five distinct phases the Fire Chi corresponds to noon (solar time) which is the period of highest Yang when we'll see the dominance in the Water Chi, the Wood Chi corresponds to the morning. The first hour of afternoon be dominated by the Earth Chi and the last hours before bed will bring on the Metal Chi.

A clear macrocosmic cycle could be the one of the tides that are controlled by the direct influence from both the Sun and Moon and, in turn, are governed by their respective cycles. Human beings, in the natural world, has the cycle of his Chi cycle and participates in the cosmic dance through being influenced by the cycles around them and then interfering with his own cycles, particularly as the global

Human Being. There are also other macrocosmic cycles, however their influence is less apparent than those of the main cycles as it is mediated through more subtle energies which like the ones we've said, are unable to create immediate and visible changes to the physical planes.

For its part, the organism of living beings maintains its own internal cycles of Yin-Yang alternation: sleep and wakefulness may be the most obvious cycle, but there is also activity-rest, food-fasting, inspiration-expiration, systole-diastole, contraction-strain, etc. The cycles of the inner universe (microcosmic) are governed by similar laws to the macrocosmic cycles. In these cycles they also have the characteristics of the Chi is also able to adopt the traits for each one of the five phases that comprise Chi Cycle. Chi Cycle.

The inner cycles of living beings (microcosms) are linked to the cycles of the entire Universe (external macrocosmic) since, without them, living beings would not be able to access the Cosmic Chi or also the Celestial Chi, without which existence would not be possible.

So, when the rising of the Sun the vast Chi of the Wood seizes us, and it energizes us all through the day. When noon arrives the body must adjust to the time when it is at its peak energy due to the effects from Fire Chi. A few minutes later, we are at the peak in the dull Chi of the Earth, and all through the afternoon, we feel its slower and reflective energies. As the Sun has already set as it is already dark and the Chi of the Metal preponderates in our body, it begins to process its energy into preparation for night, during when it is the Chi of the Water adds us to the silence. The same influence is felt throughout the season's cycle.

The external and internal cycles work together and balance each other through complex interactions. Sometimes, they are evident, but sometimes difficult to comprehend.

Conclusion

There is a Sanskrit word Chakra can be interpreted to mean "wheel" or "turning" and, even though it originated with Hindu writings, it can be used in Tibetan, Chinese, and Tamil dialects as well. Chakras Chakras are vortices that are present in our bodies . They control many aspects of our lives. even though various frameworks and numbers are in existence they are the most well-known of them have seven notable energy centers.

The Hindi writings, also known as Tantras The Chakras are depicted as Sat-Cakra-Nirupama and Padaka-Pan are part of a nebulous framework that includes the Kundalini as well. The majority of these ancient writings come in diverse forms, with a frequency between five to twelve basic Padaka-Pancakes. Nevertheless, every one of these frameworks serves one common goal: the awakening of the Kundalini by the ascent to the Chakras.

When the Kundalini is agitated and rises up through the body, it keeps to pierce the unique vortices and the individual achieves another level of Siddhi or pristine. The final goal of mindfulness is achieved at the point that the Kundalini attains the head and the person is reunited to the Divine.

Apart from those seven main Chakras smaller ones, also known as medians, are also present If any of the Chakras have not been adjusted an individual may experience negative consequences of dysfunctional or physical behavior or irregularities. The arrangement and the stimulation of these vortices may be achieved by the feeling of touch. This is the reason why those Tantric massages beneficial. When you are with an Tantric Goddess, you will not only create a new connection and receive a very sensual back rub, but additionally get the full recovery benefits too. Since Universal energy, love, and the process of learning run in our physical bodies allowing them to move freely and without difficulty is crucial for every aspect that we live.

Understanding this mind-blowing theory or being a committed follower will bring many amazing benefits. You can also use Tantric back rubs, techniques or Tantric massages methods or methods to achieve an inner harmony and agreement regardless of whether you're in any way familiar with the otherworldly aspects of this fascinating education and life reasoning.

www.ingramcontent.com/pod-product-compliance
Lightning Source LLC
Chambersburg PA
CBHW071839080526
44589CB00012B/1047